AIDS

A guide to current knowledge and prosp

AIDS

A guide to current knowledge and prospects for control

Brian Jones

HONG KONG UNIVERSITY PRESS

Printed in Hong Kong by Golden Cup Printing Company Limited

Contents

Preface

The statistics of the world-wide AIDS epidemic are horrifying, and yet here in Hong Kong, with just a trickle of cases to date, it may be hard to imagine that our society could soon be seriously threatened by this dreadful disease. AIDS is spreading fast and is making serious inroads into the general population. It can no longer be considered a disease mainly affecting gay men or drug addicts, and it is certainly not a disease against which Asians have a particular resistance.

This booklet is an attempt to summarize briefly current knowledge about the causation, symptoms, transmission, diagnosis and global spread of AIDS. The prospects for development of vaccines and successful therapy are also discussed. A thumb-nail sketch of the basic workings of the immune system is included as an appendix. Hopefully this information will be useful to medical personnel – doctors, nurses and technicians – who will increasingly be seeing patients or handling body fluids infected with the AIDS virus. Hopefully also it will be consulted by secondary school science teachers, in whose hands lies much responsibility for ensuring that young people are informed about AIDS and its prevention.

I am most grateful to the Medical Faculty and the Pathology Department, University of Hong Kong, for subsidizing the publication of this book. Also, my sincere thanks go to Anthony Yiu of the Medical Illustration Unit, University of Hong Kong and Ian Jones for the illustrations, Yvette Chow for expertly typing the manuscript, and Prof. Brian Weatherhead for particularly useful comments and suggestions.

B.M. Jones
Senior Hospital Immunologist
University of Hong Kong

July 1989

Chapter 1

What Causes AIDS?

Human immunodeficiency virus (HIV)

The acquired immunodeficiency syndrome (AIDS) is the most serious epidemic disease of modern times. It is caused by a newly discovered virus named human immunodeficiency virus (HIV), whose basic structure is shown in Fig. 1. HIV is a spherical virus of 100 nm diameter, with a surface envelope consisting of lipid and glycoprotein. A transmembrane glycoprotein, gp41 (the number refers to the approximate molecular weight in kilodaltons), is embedded in the lipid bilayer, while the gp120 glycoprotein projects externally. The core consists of two major proteins, p18 and p24, within which are two strands of ribonucleic acid (RNA) and several

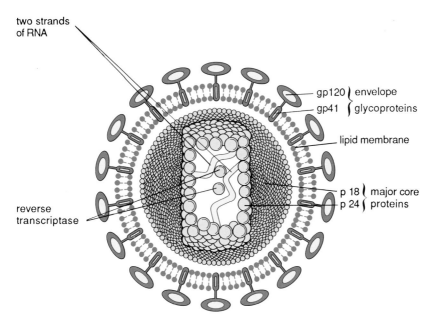

Figure 1. Structure of HIV.

molecules of an enzyme called reverse transcriptase. Within the infected host cell, the viral RNA genetic code will be converted by reverse transcriptase into a deoxyribonucleic acid (DNA) copy, and this will become incorporated into the DNA of the host cell (see next section).

Infection of T4-positive cells

HIV can bind to and infect only those human cells which have a molecule called T4* on their surface. This molecule is found in abundance primarily on helper T-lymphocytes, the central and crucial cell involved in the body's protective immune system[+]. It is the destruction of this population of cells by HIV that causes AIDS.

The T4 molecule forms a receptor for HIV on the surface of T-helper cells. HIV's gp120 fits into T4 like a key into a lock, enabling the virus to become closely associated with the helper cell. The virus' RNA then passes into the helper cell, reverse transcriptase converts the RNA into DNA, and the latter combines with the DNA of the infected cell (Fig. 2). At this stage, no harm befalls the T-helper cell, which is said to be 'latently infected'.

Destruction of T4-positive cells

If a latently-infected T-helper cell becomes activated during the course of a normal immunological reaction[+], the virus DNA is triggered to begin making all the protein components required for assembly of HIV, and thousands of copies of the virus are produced within each infected cell. When the virus particles are released, the T-helper cell is destroyed (Fig. 2).

Only a tiny proportion (approximately 1 in 10,000) of T4-positive cells in infected persons contain HIV. Since AIDS is characterized by extreme depletion of the T4-positive population, other mechanisms besides direct killing of infected cells by HIV must occur. Two such mechanisms are described in the following sections.

---

*   The more up-to-date term for this molecule is 'CD4', however T4 is used throughout this booklet as it may be more familiar to readers.

+   See Appendix.

(1) HIV binds to T4 on the surface of T-helper lymphocytes via gp120.

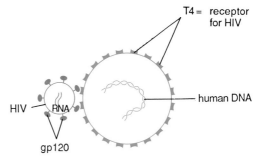

T-helper lymphocyte

(2) HIV enters target cell, leaving gp120 molecules on the surface. Virus RNA is converted to DNA by reverse transcriptase. Virus DNA is incorporated into host cell genes.

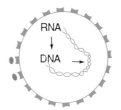

Latently-infected T-helper lymphocyte

(3) An immunological stimulus triggers rapid transcription and translation of viral DNA into HIV proteins. Thousands of new virus particles bud from the T-helper lymphocyte surface.

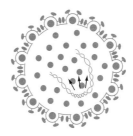

T-helper lymphocyte destroyed

Figure 2. Infection and destruction of T-helper lymphocytes.

Giant cells

HIV-infected T-helper cells can bind to other, uninfected, helper cells via surface membrane gp120, following which adjacent cell membranes become fused together and 'giant cells' are formed. The entire giant cell is destroyed when virus particles are released (Fig. 3). In this way HIV is able to pass from cell to cell within the body without ever being exposed to potentially neutralizing antibodies or killer cells.

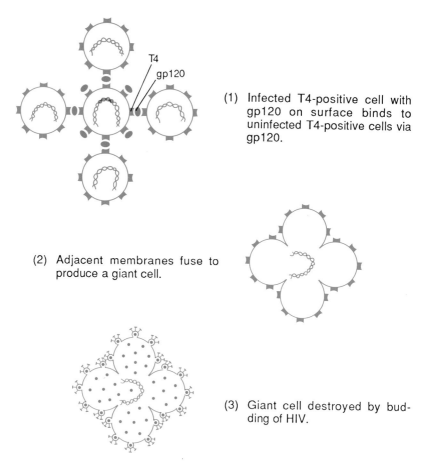

(1) Infected T4-positive cell with gp120 on surface binds to uninfected T4-positive cells via gp120.

(2) Adjacent membranes fuse to produce a giant cell.

(3) Giant cell destroyed by budding of HIV.

Figure 3. Formation of giant cells.

Autoimmune destruction of T4-positive cells

T-helper cells can also be destroyed by the very immune system products which were induced during the body's first encounter with HIV. This is because infected T-helper cells can release molecules of HIV gp120 from their surface, and these bind to T4 on other, uninfected, T-helper cells. These are recognized and destroyed by antibodies and killer cells reactive with gp120 (Fig. 4).

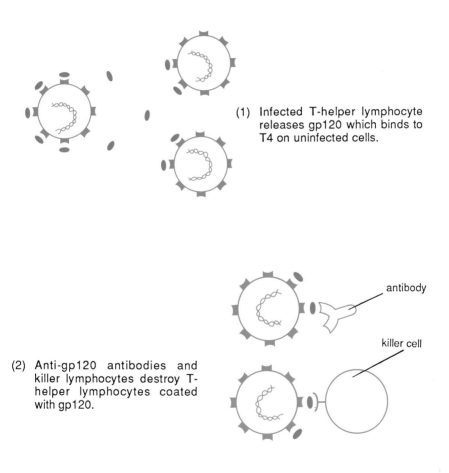

(1) Infected T-helper lymphocyte releases gp120 which binds to T4 on uninfected cells.

antibody

killer cell

(2) Anti-gp120 antibodies and killer lymphocytes destroy T-helper lymphocytes coated with gp120.

Figure 4. Autoimmune destruction of T-helper lymphocytes.

Infection of macrophages

The T4-positive helper cell population is undoubtably the primary target for HIV, but certain other cells in the body, notably scavenger cells called macrophages, also carry small numbers of T4 molecules on their surface and can be infected by HIV. Macrophages probably do not support proliferation of HIV, but they serve as a reservoir for the virus and are responsible for transporting HIV to the brain. The normal functions of macrophages, clearing the body of debris and 'presenting' antigen to T-helper lymphocytes, are severely inhibited following infection with HIV.

Chapter 2

What are the Symptoms of HIV Infection?

Acute illness and the carrier state

Approximately two to four weeks after initial infection with HIV, many (but not all) subjects suffer an acute influenza- or mononucleosis-like illness from which they recover rapidly (Fig. 5). Antibodies against HIV appear at between 3 weeks and 3 months (sometimes longer). At this stage the subject is a latently infected carrier of HIV: the viral DNA is incorporated into the DNA of a small number of T4-positive helper cells and macrophages, but there is little proliferation of the virus, the immune system is intact and there are no disease symptoms. The subject is, however, infectious, and could unknowingly transmit the virus to others.

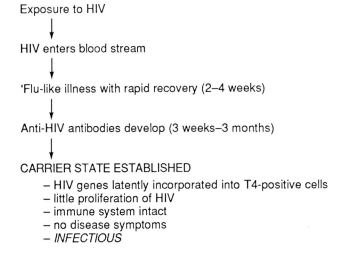

Exposure to HIV

↓

HIV enters blood stream

↓

'Flu-like illness with rapid recovery (2–4 weeks)

↓

Anti-HIV antibodies develop (3 weeks–3 months)

↓

CARRIER STATE ESTABLISHED
- HIV genes latently incorporated into T4-positive cells
- little proliferation of HIV
- immune system intact
- no disease symptoms
- *INFECTIOUS*

Figure 5. Early stages of HIV infection.

Lymphadenopathy syndrome

Eventually an infected T-helper cell receives an immunological stimulus and this triggers a wave of virus proliferation (see page 2) which leads to a gradual destruction of the T-helper population. As this population becomes depleted, immunological defences become weaker and symptoms of disease become more severe (Fig. 6). Initially the only sign of HIV infection is enlargement of lymph glands in various parts of the body (lymphadenopathy syndrome): this represents the body's struggle to respond immunologically against the virus. This stage may last for months or years, but progression to more severe disease now seems to be inevitable.

AIDS-related complex (ARC)

ARC is characterized by the appearance of constitutional symptoms, such as prolonged fever, severe weight loss, diarrhoea, fatigue, night sweats and the first real sign of immune deficiency – oral *Candida* infection (thrush).

AIDS

As the T-helper cell count drops and the patient becomes severely immunodeficient, aggressive infections (notably pneumonia due to *Pneumocystis carinii*) and/or malignancies (Kaposi's sarcoma, lymphoma) signal the arrival of full-blown AIDS (Fig. 7).

Neurological disease

Many AIDS victims also suffer neurological disease – encephalitis and/or dementia – resulting from infection of the brain by HIV itself or by other pathogens, and indeed HIV-induced neurological disease may be the earliest or only manifestation of AIDS.

Death

80% of AIDS patients die within 2 years of diagnosis, the median survival time being less than one year.

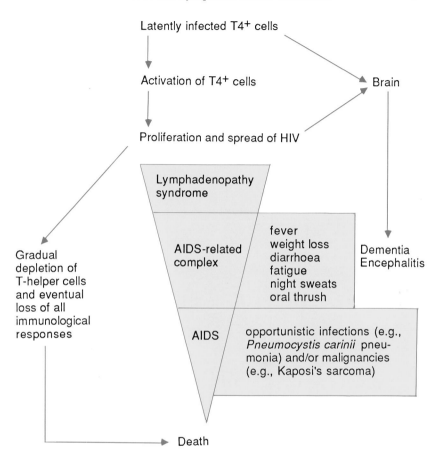

Figure 6. Development of disease.

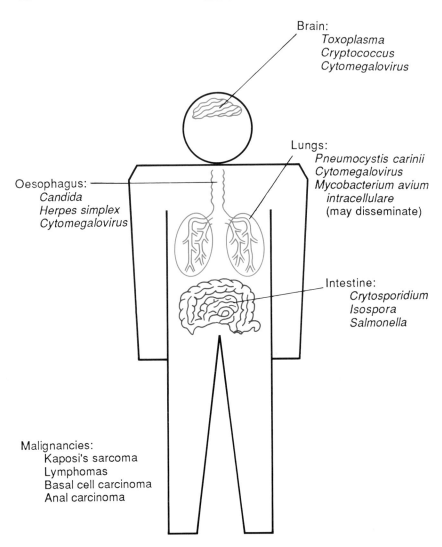

Brain:
  Toxoplasma
  Cryptococcus
  Cytomegalovirus

Lungs:
  Pneumocystis carinii
  Cytomegalovirus
  Mycobacterium avium
  intracellulare
  (may disseminate)

Oesophagus: —
  Candida
  Herpes simplex
  Cytomegalovirus

Intestine:
  Crytosporidium
  Isospora
  Salmonella

Malignancies:
  Kaposi's sarcoma
  Lymphomas
  Basal cell carcinoma
  Anal carcinoma

Figure 7. Infections and malignancies in AIDS.

Chapter 3

How is HIV Transmitted?

Routes of transmission of HIV are summarized in Table 1.

Table 1. Routes of transmission of HIV.

1. Sexual
   - male-to-male
   - male-to-female
   - female-to-male

2. Injection
   - blood transfusion
   - blood products, notably Factor VIII (haemophiliacs)
   - sharing blood–contaminated needles and syringes (addicts who inject drugs)

3. Mother to infant
   - across placenta
   - breast-feeding*

Casual contact, eg., kissing, hugging, sharing bathroom or eating facilities, caring for AIDS patients, does *not* transmit HIV.

* Few documented cases.

Sexual transmission

The major route of transmission of HIV is by heterosexual or homosexual intercourse. For transmission to occur, live, infectious virus must be present in the semen or vaginal fluid of one partner and gain access to the blood stream of the other. Cell-free virus is poorly infectious, so in effect T4-positive cells that are infected with HIV must be transmitted. Such cells are present in genital secretions of HIV carriers.

Other sexually transmitted diseases (STDs)

Sexual transmission of HIV is enhanced in the presence of other STDs such as gonorrhoea or syphilis, because (a) the genital secretions of STD patients contain raised numbers of T4-positive cells, and (b) genital lesions permit easier entry of HIV. Thus sexual intercourse is most dangerous when performed with a promiscuous partner, since the higher the number of sexual partners, the higher is the risk of exposure to HIV *and* to other STDs.

Condoms

Undamaged latex condoms are an effective barrier against transmission of STDs, including HIV infection. They must, however, be used correctly (Table 2), and it is recommended that they be used in conjunction with a spermicide which contains nonoxynol-9, a powerful inactivator of HIV.

Table 2. Correct use of condoms.

- Use a good quality electronically-tested *latex* condom of the correct size; 'natural' condoms made from sheep intestine do not prevent the passage of HIV.

- Use a condom every time you have intercourse with someone who *could* carry HIV.

- Put the condom on as soon as erection occurs.

- Roll the condom's rim all the way to the base of the penis. If the condom lacks a reservoir tip, leave a small space at the tip to catch semen.

- Do not use petroleum jelly, vegetable oil or saliva for lubrication – they can damage latex. Water can be used, but a spermicidal jelly or foam containing nonoxynol-9 (which inactivates HIV) is recommended.

- After ejaculation, withdraw the penis immediately, holding on to the rim of the condom.

- Do not use a condom more than once. Dispose of it safely.

- Store condoms in a cool, dry place. Do not keep them in a wallet or other hot places as this may damage the latex.

Anal and vaginal sex

A recent Australian study has attempted to determine the relative efficiency of HIV transmission by various forms of sexual activity (Table 3). Recipients of anal intercourse became infected about twice as often as recipients of vaginal intercourse when exposed on the same number of occasions to HIV-infected men. Female to male transmission during vaginal intercourse was about half as efficient as from male to female.

Table 3.   Comparison of HIV transmission rates by anal and vaginal intercourse.

HIV was transmitted following 10–50 episodes of sexual intercourse with an HIV-infected partner in:

1. 37–48% of men or women exposed by receptive anal intercourse

2. 20–28% of women exposed by receptive vaginal intercourse

3. 10–13% of men exposed by insertive vaginal intercourse

(Data from J.M. Dwyer, presented at 1st International Congress on AIDS in Asia, November 1987)

Blood transfusion

HIV is readily transmitted by intravenous injection of HIV-infected blood, or blood products such as clotting factors used in the treatment of haemophilia. This form of transmission is now largely preventable, since all blood donors can be screened by sensitive tests for HIV infection (see later). However, these tests rely on measurement of antibodies against HIV, and as already discussed, antibodies are not present until at least 3 weeks after exposure to the virus. Thus it is vital that persons who *could* have been exposed to HIV refrain from donating blood.

Intravenous drug abuse

A major route of transmission of HIV is amongst intravenous drug abusers who share drug injection equipment. Sharing of needles and syringes may often be due to shortage of supply, but an emotional need to experience closeness or togetherness is another factor. It is proving to be extremely difficult to encourage changes of behaviour in this group: needle exchange programmes and advice to sterilize needles and syringes with bleach before use are not reducing the rate at which intravenous drug abusers are becoming infected with HIV. Sexual partners of drug addicts are at high risk of HIV infection, and the potential exists for widespread transmission of HIV by addicts who support their habit by prostitution.

Neonatal transmission

Approximately half of all pregnant women infected with HIV give birth to infected babies. Infection probably occurs across the placenta rather than at the time of delivery, because babies delivered by Caesarian section do not escape infection. HIV infection progresses rapidly in infants, and pregnancy may accelerate development of AIDS in the mother.

Breast-feeding

HIV has been isolated from breast milk and there has been some concern that breast-feeding could transmit the virus. However there have been few documented cases of this happening: in one case the mother became infected with HIV by blood transfusion given *after* the baby had been delivered, and the breast-fed baby eventually tested positive for HIV antibodies. In this case HIV probably entered through the skin (the baby had severe eczema) rather than via the digestive tract. In those parts of the world where nutritionally sufficient human milk substitutes are available and can be hygienically prepared, mothers who are known HIV carriers are advised not to breast-feed. However in poorer developing countries the risk of the baby becoming infected with HIV by breast-feeding is considered to be far less than the risk of malnutrition or infectious disease if breast-feeding is withheld.

Casual contact

In a tiny number of cases, HIV has been transmitted to health-care personnel, but since tens of thousands of doctors, nurses and laboratory workers are knowingly or unknowingly in contact with HIV carriers, this argues strongly against transmission by casual contact. The documented cases of transmission to health-care workers have involved either accidental injury with needles attached to syringes containing HIV-infected blood, during the course of which patient's blood was injected into the recipient, or splashes of contaminated body fluids or concentrated virus to mouth, eyes or damaged skin.

The extreme rarity of transmission of HIV to household contacts of infected persons again indicates that transmission does not normally occur by routes other than sexual intercourse, injection, or from mother to child in the womb. Normal affectionate behaviour, including kissing and hugging, does not transmit HIV, nor does sharing bathroom facilities, nor does sharing eating or drinking utensils.

Chapter 4

Testing for HIV Infection

Screening of blood donations

In most developed countries, all blood donations are now screened for antibodies against HIV, the presence of which indicates that the donor has been exposed to the virus and that use of the blood for transfusion would endanger the recipient. An enzyme-linked immunosorbent assay (ELISA) is used to test for HIV antibodies. This test is extremely sensitive and the chance of a positive sample being missed by an experienced laboratory is low. The test is not quite so specific, and approximately 0.2% of samples give a 'false positive' result. It is therefore essential to re-test all positive samples by a different ELISA system, and if confirmed as ELISA-positive, to test yet again using a more specific test such as Western blot, immunofluorescence or radioimmune precipitation. Only then should the blood donor be informed that he or she is a likely carrier of HIV.

Alternative testing sites

The danger exists that persons who participate in risky behaviour, such as casual sexual relationships or intravenous drug abuse, might attempt to donate blood in order to determine their HIV status. Although such donations would be screened by the highly sensitive ELISA test, infected blood could test negative if the donor had been exposed to HIV only recently. This is because antibodies to HIV do not appear until 3 weeks to 3 months (sometimes longer) after infection. These blood donations would of course be likely to infect their recipients. Testing sites other than blood transfusion units, such as STD clinics or virology laboratories, are therefore available in most developed countries, and usually the test can be arranged through general practitioners.

ELISA for HIV antigens

New ELISA tests that measure the presence of HIV *antigen* in blood have recently been developed, and these are able to identify infected persons as little as 2 weeks after exposure. However, because of the great expense of performing this test on all donated blood samples, and because relatively few additional positive samples would be identified, the HIV antigen ELISA has not gained acceptance as an additional screening test.

HIV serology and disease progression

HIV antigen can be demonstrated in blood early after exposure, but its level rapidly declines when antibodies appear (Fig. 8). Antibodies are formed against all the components of the virus, those directed against the envelope are usually present throughout the life of the patient, but those that react with core proteins decline and eventually disappear when the disease becomes severe. When anti-core antibodies disappear, HIV antigen rises to high levels. An infected subject is most infectious when HIV antigen levels are high, i.e., soon after infection (when he or she could be unaware that infection has occurred) and after development of severe disease.

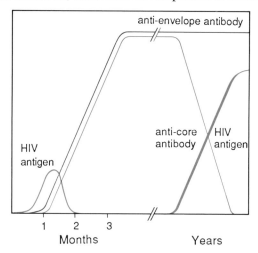

Figure 8. HIV serology and disease progression.

HIV serology and the origin of HIV

The ELISA for HIV antibodies has been used to investigate the time and place of origin of HIV, using serum samples from many parts of the world which had been stored frozen for many years. One sample collected in 1959 from a patient in Kinshasa, Zaire, tested positive for HIV antibodies, but it is possible that this isolated result was a false positive, because after prolonged storage this specimen became very sticky and could have adhered non-specifically to the HIV antigens used in the ELISA.

Fifty out of 75 samples collected from clinically healthy persons in a rural community in Uganda in 1972 were found to contain HIV antibodies, suggesting that infection with HIV or a virtually identical virus was present and widespread in Central Africa long before AIDS was recognized in the developed world. It remains very much a mystery as to why none of these Ugandan blood donors exhibited symptoms of HIV infection; possibly HIV has subsequently undergone subtle changes which have increased its virulence, alternatively members of this rural community may have developed a natural immunity against the virus.

Chapter 5

The World-wide Spread of AIDS

When did the epidemic begin?

AIDS was first recognized as a new clinical entity in the summer of 1981, at which time physicians in New York and San Francisco began to notice an unprecedented number of young men presenting with either aggressive Kaposi's sarcoma or *Pneumocystis carinii* pneumonia, diseases which are extremely uncommon except in severely immunocompromised patients.

The cause of this new syndrome was not known until late 1983, when Prof. Luc Montagnier of the Pasteur Institute, Paris and later Dr. Robert Gallo of the National Cancer Institute, Bethesda, independently isolated the virus that we now call HIV. ELISA's for measuring HIV antibodies were developed in 1985.

Although AIDS was not actually recognized until 1981, retrospective analysis of case reports has indicated that the disease has been occurring in Central Africa since 1976 and in the United States since 1978. The first AIDS cases in Europe were reported in 1980 and in Australasia and Asia in 1983.

What is the extent of the epidemic?

The World Health Organization estimates that there have been 200,000–250,000 cases of AIDS world-wide up to the time of writing (July 1988) (Table 4). The highest number of cases is presumed to be in sub-Saharan Africa, though accurate figures are difficult to obtain from this region due to primitive diagnostic and reporting facilities and frequently erroneous diagnosis of AIDS as malnutrition or parasitic infection. The Americas have almost 75,000 cases (more than 65,000 from USA), Europe over 12,000, Australasia almost 1,000 and Asia over 200. At the present time, 13 cases of AIDS have been diagnosed in Hong Kong and there are only two survivors. An additional 109 HIV carriers have been identified here. Approximately half of the known carriers in Hong Kong were infected by blood products prior to the development of screening tests for donated blood; most of the rest were infected by male homosexual activity.

Table 4. Numbers of AIDS cases by continent, mid 1988.

Africa	11,753*
USA	65,099
The Americas, excluding USA	9,763
Europe	12,594
Australasia	956
Asia	243
TOTAL	100,408+
Hong Kong	122 HIV-infected persons 13 AIDS cases 11 deaths

*   In Africa, the reported number of AIDS cases grossly underestimates the true prevalence.
+   W.H.O. estimates 200,000–250,000 AIDS cases world-wide.

Numbers of ARC cases

AIDS-related complex is approximately five times more prevalent than AIDS itself, and the total number of ARC cases is estimated to be more than 1 million. Progression from ARC to AIDS occurs at a rate of approximately 10% per year, and it is expected that virtually all of the present ARC cases will eventually develop AIDS.

Numbers of HIV carriers

The number of symptom-free HIV carriers is believed to exceed the number of AIDS cases by a factor of 50–100. Thus between 10 and 25 million people world-wide are thought to be infected with HIV. No definite statements can be made as to how many of the carriers will eventually develop serious symptoms, nor is the median length of the latency period known. However a recent study performed in San Francisco reported that 74% of HIV-infected male homosexuals progressed to ARC or AIDS over a 7-year observation period. It is now generally believed that the great majority of HIV carriers will eventually develop AIDS.

Projections for the future

Since the beginning of the epidemic, the number of AIDS cases has been doubling approximately every 12 months. Thus it can be projected that by 1991, 10 years after the recognized start of the epidemic, there will have been between 1 and 2 million cases of AIDS, 5–10 million ARC cases, and 80–200 million persons will be carriers of HIV (Fig. 9).

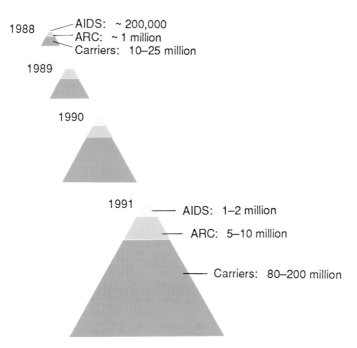

Figure 9. Projected growth of the epidemic.

Can we reduce the spread of AIDS?

Considerable progress has been made towards developing vaccines for prevention of AIDS (see later) but this urgent objective is still many years away. Certain anti-viral drugs have been developed which may prolong survival of AIDS patients (again, see later) but these are still too toxic to be taken for life. We are left with the stark realization that at present we are powerless to prevent the development of HIV disease in the 10–25 million persons now thought to be infected with HIV.

Can we, though, prevent *further* spread of HIV and so prevent the dreadful possibility of 80–200 million carriers by 1991? Our only available weapon against AIDS is education of all sectors of society about the nature of the disease and its transmission.

Examples of succinct messages which could serve to underline certain aspects of HIV transmission are given in Table 5.

Table 5. AIDS educational messages.

– 'AIDS spreads FAST but kills SLOW.'
– 'Casual sex is RISKY (condoms give some protection).'
– 'If you share works* you could share AIDS.'
– 'Don't get pregnant if you could get AIDS.'
– 'AIDS – a world-wide effort will stop it.'+

* drug injection equipment
+ slogan of the World Health Organization

High risk groups

In the developed countries of North America, Europe and Australia, AIDS is associated with certain high risk behaviour, notably male homosexual intercourse and intravenous drug abuse (Table 6). A notable feature of the AIDS epidemic has been the positive response of the homosexual community to advice to change behaviour in order to reduce transmission, and this has resulted in a reducing trend in the proportion of AIDS cases contracted as a result of male homosexual activity. This has not been the case amongst intravenous drug abusers, whose representation among AIDS cases is continuing to rise. The percentage of cases associated with blood transfusion and treatment with clotting factors for haemophilia are gradually decreasing as a result of the introduction of tests for screening blood donors. Conversely, the proportion of cases associated with heterosexual transmission is increasing.

Table 6. Adult AIDS cases by risk factor — USA.

Homosexual/bisexual male	65.7%
IV drug abuser	16.6%
Homosexual and drug abuser	7.6%
Heterosexual partner	3.9%
Haemophilia/blood transfusion	3.2%
Unknown	3.0%

The tragedy of Africa

In Africa AIDS is known as 'slim disease' and it is endemic in many Central African countries (Fig. 10). Male homosexuality and intravenous drug abuse have not been the major factors in the development of the epidemic. AIDS occurs in almost equal numbers of men and women, and undoubtably the principal routes of transmission have been heterosexual intercourse, blood transfusion and transmission from mother to the developing foetus.

A number of factors has led to the explosion of AIDS cases in Central Africa. One has been the change from a mainly rural, agricultural way of life to an increasingly urbanized society. HIV may once have existed only in small rural communities in Africa (see Chapter 4), and could have become more widely disseminated after migration to the towns. Whether this is the case or not, urbanization undoubtedly created greater opportunities for promiscuity: husbands leaving wives and families to seek employment in urban areas would have availed themselves of prostitutes for sexual gratification; deserted wives may have turned to prostitution to support children and families. That this could have caused rapid dissemination of HIV is indicated by the high prevalence of HIV infection amongst African prostitutes (eg., 88% of prostitutes in Rwanda are HIV carriers).

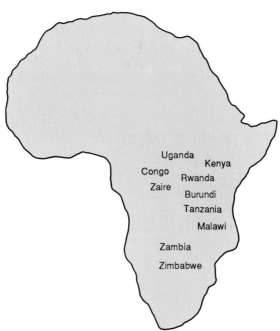

Figure 10. Countries in Africa most severely affected by AIDS.

A second major factor in Africa is the extremely limited funds available for health care. In many Central African countries blood for transfusion is usually not screened for HIV antibodies, and since up to 15% of blood donors have been found to carry HIV, transmission by this route is alarmingly high. Transfusion of blood is rather commonplace in Africa where malaria, which causes anaemia, is endemic. Inadequate health budgets also lead to the common practice of re-using medical equipment such as needles, syringes and scalpels, with the consequent possibility of transmitting HIV.

A number of studies have shown that the prevalence of HIV infection in pregnant women in Central Africa is very high, up to 15 % in certain cities. At least half of the babies born to these women will themselves be infected with HIV.

The tragedy of Africa will continue unless governments of developed countries provide massive financial assistance. The tragedy of Africa must not be allowed to occur elsewhere.

Chapter 6

Vaccines for AIDS

Special problems posed by HIV

Remarkable progress has been made in understanding the nature of the virus that causes AIDS since its isolation just 5 years ago. Most notably, HIV's genetic organization is now reasonably well understood, and the exact sequence of the approximately 10,000 nucleotides that make up the virus' genes is known for several different HIV isolates*. This work has revealed that it will be extremely difficult to develop a simple vaccine against HIV, because nucleotide sequences, and hence the amino acid sequences of the proteins they encode, vary significantly between different HIV isolates. The amino acid sequence of HIV's envelope (the primary target for the immune system and hence a logical candidate for a vaccine) may vary by as much as 20% from isolate to isolate. Thus a vaccine prepared from one isolate of HIV may not protect against all the different forms of the virus. Furthermore, HIV appears to be able to subtly alter its structure in the body, a process known as 'antigenic drift'. This may allow the virus to escape destruction by the immune system.

Despite these problems, research into HIV vaccines is progressing along several different avenues, and there are hopes that safe and effective vaccines will eventually be produced which will induce protective antibodies in those at risk but not yet infected with HIV, and which will activate killer lymphocytes able to destroy infected T-helper lymphocytes in those already infected.

Synthetic polypeptide vaccines

Although the overall structure of HIV's envelope varies widely between different isolates, certain regions within the envelope seem

---

* To obtain an HIV isolate, lymphocytes from the patient are incubated with special T4-positive cancer cells called H9, which support proliferation of HIV without themselves being killed. Sufficient material can be obtained to analyse that isolate's nucleotide sequence.

to be identical, or nearly so, for all known isolates. For example, a conserved polypeptide consisting of amino acids 735–752 was identified by computer analysis of nucleotide sequences of envelope genes from several HIV isolates. This polypeptide (Fig. 11) has been synthesized and used to immunize rabbits, and these produced antibodies which prevented the growth of HIV in cultured T-helper lymphocytes.

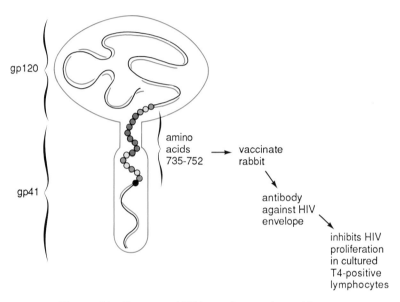

Figure 11. Conserved HIV envelope polypeptide.

Recombinant vaccines

The recombinant DNA technology can be used to obtain large quantities of any required protein, provided the gene for that protein can be identified and isolated. The HIV envelope gene has been so obtained and has been introduced into the genome of a bacterium (*Escherichia coli*). When the modified *E. coli* is grown in laboratory culture, it synthesizes large amounts of HIV envelope protein which can be readily purified from the culture fluid (Fig. 12). The recombinant envelope protein induces antibodies in immunized animals which neutralize HIV, and it is currently being tested for toxicity and immunogenicity in a small group of human volunteers.

The HIV envelope gene has also been introduced into the genome of vaccinia virus (the attenuated virus used in vaccination against smallpox). Experimental animals, and subsequently a small group of human volunteers, were vaccinated with this live recombinant vaccine and they developed antibodies which neutralized not only the isolate of HIV from which the envelope gene was originally prepared, but also several other HIV isolates of widely differing envelope structure. Particularly encouraging was the development of activated lymphocytes able to kill HIV-infected T-helper lymphocytes by one of the human volunteers who received several booster doses of the vaccine.

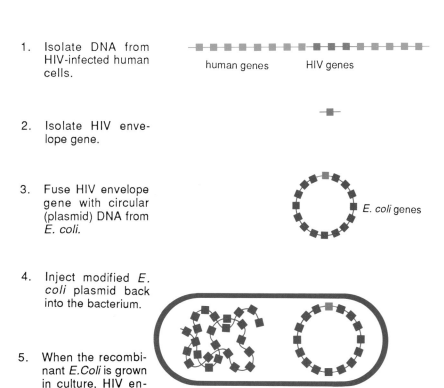

1. Isolate DNA from HIV-infected human cells.

human genes   HIV genes

2. Isolate HIV envelope gene.

3. Fuse HIV envelope gene with circular (plasmid) DNA from E. coli.

E. coli genes

4. Inject modified E. coli plasmid back into the bacterium.

5. When the recombinant E.Coli is grown in culture, HIV envelope protein will be produced in addition to normal E. Coli products.

Figure 12. Recombinant HIV envelope vaccine.

Killed whole virus vaccines

Boosting the antibody response of patients with early signs of HIV infection might reduce the rate of progression to full-blown AIDS. This is being tested in a small trial using whole HIV killed by irradiation.

Attenuated virus vaccines

Since live virus vaccines generally produce a stronger cell-mediated immune response than killed virus vaccines, the possibility that HIV could be attenuated by altering or removing certain of its genes is now being investigated. HIV is similar to other retroviruses in possessing 'gag' genes which specify core proteins, 'pol' genes which specify reverse transcriptase, and 'env' genes specifying the envelope, but in addition has certain unique genes responsible for pathogenicity ('tat' – transactivator of transcription, '3'orf' – open reading frame, 'art' – anti-repressor of transactivation and 'sor' – short open reading frame) (Fig. 13). Deletion mutants of HIV,

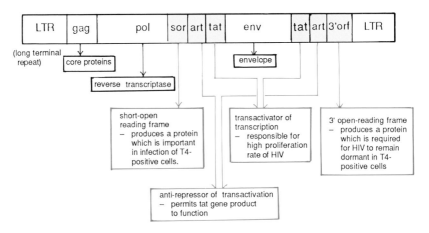

Genes shown in red are responsible for HIV's pathogenicity. Attenuated vaccines could be produced by deleting some of these genes.

Figure 13. Genetic organization of HIV.

lacking certain of these 'pathogenic' genes, have been prepared, and these mutants proliferate poorly or not at all in cultured human T4-positive lymphocytes. They do, however, stimulate an immune response against HIV when injected into animals.

Limited trials of attenuated HIV vaccines are now being contemplated in human volunteers, but first it is necessary to be certain that the deletion mutants cannot revert to a pathogenic form in the body.

Anti-idiotype vaccines

A totally different and novel approach to producing vaccines uses anti-idiotype antibodies (anti-antibodies) to mimic immunogenic structures of pathogens (Fig. 14). The idiotype of an antibody

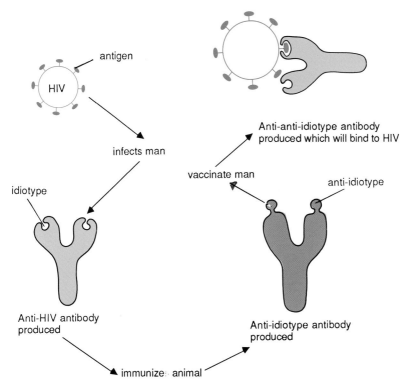

Figure 14. Anti-idiotype vaccine.

is the part of the molecule that actually binds to the antigen, and has a molecular configuration which is the mirror image of the antigen, allowing the antigen to fit into the idiotype like a key into a lock. Purified idiotype is itself immunogenic and will induce anti-idiotype antibodies when injected into an animal. The molecular configuration of the anti-idiotype is the mirror image of the idiotype, and thus will closely resemble the shape of the original antigen.

Antibodies against HIV obtained from naturally infected persons have been purified and used to vaccinate mice. Purified anti-idiotype antibodies mimic HIV antigens and could be injected into humans as a surrogate for HIV antigens. This approach would be free of the inherent risks of injecting antigens prepared from HIV.

Trials of candidate vaccines

The only species apart from man that can be infected with HIV is the chimpanzee, and these animals do not develop symptoms of AIDS. Chimpanzees are an endangered species, and only small numbers are available for testing candidate vaccines for the ability to protect against challenge with live HIV.

In the absence of a suitable animal model for AIDS*, several research groups have proceeded to limited trials of HIV vaccines in human volunteers. Obviously no vaccinated volunteer could be knowingly challenged with live HIV to discover whether or not protective immunity had been developed, and it will only be possible to evaluate efficacy of candidate vaccines by comparing infection rates of members of high risk groups who have or have not been vaccinated. This information will take many years to accumulate.

---

* Recent months have seen major progress in developing animal models for HIV infection in species other than chimpanzees, and these should certainly expedite the development of effective vaccines and therapies.

Chapter 7

Therapy for AIDS

Prevention of HIV proliferation

It is most unlikely that HIV infected persons could be rendered virus-free by treatment with drugs, because latent virus within T4-positive cells cannot be destroyed without also destroying the host cells. Instead a major effort has been made to develop drugs which could prevent proliferation of HIV, since if this could be achieved, destruction of T-helper lymphocytes and development of immunodeficiency would be slowed or halted. Since inhibitors of HIV proliferation would have to be taken for life by HIV carriers, it is vital that they interfere with proliferation of the virus but not the host cells, and are free of toxic side effects.

A sensitive culture technique has been used to test literally thousands of chemicals for anti-HIV activity. Human T4-positive cells are infected with HIV and stimulated immunologically to induce virus proliferation. Reverse transcriptase concentrations are measured in the culture supernatant each day and drugs that reduce the amount of reverse transcriptase produced can be identified (Fig. 15). Among the drugs found to be active in this system are: Ribavirin, which has previously been used to treat a tropical virus disease known as Lassa fever; Suramin, used in the treatment of trypanosomiasis; HPA-23, an antimoniotungstate compound developed for experimental treatment of AIDS; and Foscarnet, an experimental drug developed for treating genital herpes. These drugs have been tested for therapeutic effect in patients with AIDS, but unfortunately no significant benefits have been demonstrated.

Zidovudine

3'azido 3'deoxythymidine (AZT, now known as Zidovudine) is the only drug so far shown to inhibit HIV proliferation in the body as well as in cultured HIV-infected T4-positive cells. This agent is an analogue of the nucleoside thymidine, one of the building blocks of

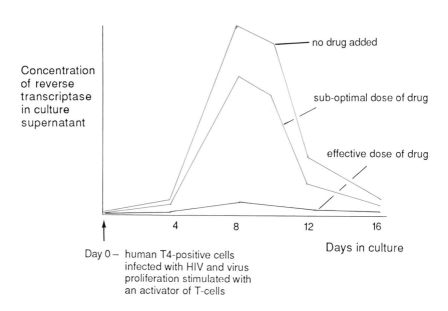

Concentration of reverse transcriptase in culture supernatant

no drug added

sub-optimal dose of drug

effective dose of drug

4   8   12   16

Days in culture

Day 0 – human T4-positive cells infected with HIV and virus proliferation stimulated with an activator of T-cells

Note: The concentration of reverse transcriptase drops after 8 days because the T4-positive cells capable of supporting HIV proliferation are all killed by the virus.

Figure 15. Inhibition of HIV proliferation by drugs.

DNA, and it is built into the growing chain of viral DNA when RNA is converted into DNA by reverse transcriptase (see p.2 and Fig. 2). This prevents elongation of the DNA chain and inhibits HIV proliferation.

In 1987 the United States Public Health Service (U.S.P.H.S.) initiated a controlled clinical trial of Zidovudine in AIDS patients who had already suffered an attack of *Pneumocystis carinii* pneumonia. Out of 145 patients treated with Zidovudine for 24 weeks, only one patient died, while in the control placebo-treated group there were 16/137 deaths (Table 7). Patients who received Zidovudine showed significantly improved counts of T4-positive lymphocytes and reduced levels of HIV antigen in the circulation, and various tests of immunologic function improved significantly. Zidovudine was found to cross the blood/brain barrier and reduce neurological symptoms of HIV infection. However many patients showed severe side effects, notably reduced numbers of red blood cells (anaemia) and neutrophils (neutropenia). These side effects could be reversed by lowering the Zidovudine dose or suspending treatment temporarily. Zidovudine is by no means a perfect treatment of HIV infection, but it is certainly the best currently available and it is now the yardstick by which new anti-HIV drugs will be judged. The major stumbling block to widespread use of Zidovudine is its price – US$8,000 per patient per year.

Table 7.   U.S. Public Health Service clinical trial of Zidovudine.

Zidovudine group :   1/145 deaths
Placebo group   :   16/137 deaths

Side effects of Zidovudine :   anaemia, neutropenia
                                                   (controllable)
Benefits of Zidovudine:
  – improved count of T4-positive lymphocytes
  – improved results in laboratory tests of immune function
  – reduced level of HIV antigen in blood
  – improved neurological signs

Zidovudine has only been tested in patients with symptomatic HIV infection, but trials will shortly begin of low, sub-toxic dosage in symptomless HIV carriers to determine whether it can prevent progression to ARC and AIDS. It is also being tested in combination with other anti-viral agents: a preliminary trial of Zidovudine plus alpha-interferon (an anti-viral agent produced naturally by virus-infected white blood cells) has shown benefits in patients with HIV-induced Kaposi's sarcoma, even with much lower doses of Zidovudine than used in the U.S.P.H.S. trial. Low dose Zidovudine has also been used in combination with another nucleoside analogue, 2'3' dideoxycytidine, with reported promising results. Dideoxycytidine could be a useful anti-HIV drug in its own right, since it is a more potent inhibitor of HIV proliferation in cultured T4-positive lymphocytes than Zidovudine and therefore could be used in treatment at lower doses with hopefully fewer side effects. A clinical trial of dideoxycytidine is now underway and the results are anxiously awaited.

Peptide-T

A different potentially useful therapeutic strategy would be to interfere with the binding of HIV to the T4 molecule on target cells. Peptide-T is a recently discovered sequence of 8 amino acids from a conserved region of gp120 which appears to be important for binding HIV to T4. Thus Peptide-T might be able to saturate HIV binding sites on T4 and prevent attachment of HIV (Fig. 16). Peptide-T protects T4-positive cells against infection with HIV in laboratory cultures (though some researchers have failed to obtain this result). A clinical trial of Peptide-T is now underway

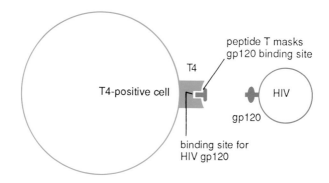

Figure 16. Peptide T inhibits binding of HIV to target cells.

Soluble T4

An alternative way of preventing the binding of HIV to T4 would be to saturate virus gp120 with soluble T4 molecules (Fig. 17). These can be produced in bulk by recombinant DNA technology (see p.28) and it has been shown that soluble T4 inhibits the infection of T4-positive cells and formation of giant cells in laboratory cultures. Clinical trials of soluble T4 are planned for the near future.

Soluble T4 molecules might even be used to kill HIV-infected T4-positive cells. Soluble T4 could be tagged with toxic agents, and these would be expected to 'home' specifically to cells bearing HIV gp120 on the membrane. Destruction of the target cells would occur if the toxins were taken up into the cytoplasm.

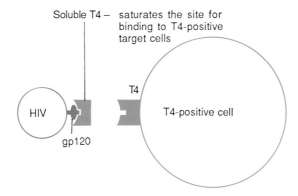

Figure 17. Soluble T4 inhibits binding of HIV to target cells.

Reconstitution of immune function

Bone marrow transplantation is the treatment of choice for repairing certain type of immunodeficiency, since bone marrow contains progenitor cells for the various cellular elements of the immune system. This therapy has been attempted in a small number of AIDS patients, and in each case partially restored immune function was achieved. However the newly induced T4-positive cells were rapidly destroyed by HIV still present in the body, and all patients died.

A major problem with bone marrow transplantation is that the donor and recipient must be precisely tissue-matched, otherwise grafted cells will either be rejected by the recipient or will attack the tissues of the recipient. The best marrow donor is a brother or sister of the patient with an identical tissue type, and since the chance of siblings being identical in this respect is only 1 in 4, few AIDS patients will have a suitable marrow donor.

A different approach to immune reconstitution which does not depend on the availability of a histocompatible donor would be to use soluble products of T-helper cells (lymphokines) and macrophages (monokines) to induce protective immune function. These are hormone-like factors which relay messages between cells of the immune system*. Their activity is extremely complex and is still the

---

* See Appendix

subject of intense investigation, but factors which promote: (a) activation of B-lymphocytes to produce antibody; (b) T-lymphocyte activation, proliferation and differentiation to killer cells; (c) macrophage and natural killer cell activation; (d) differentiation of bone marrow progenitor cells to mature cells of the immune system; and (e) destruction of tumour cells, have been identified. Several lymphokines and monokines have been produced in large quantities by recombinant DNA technology and could be evaluated in clinical trials.

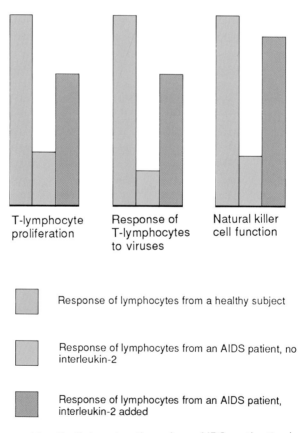

| T-lymphocyte proliferation | Response of T-lymphocytes to viruses | Natural killer cell function |

Response of lymphocytes from a healthy subject

Response of lymphocytes from an AIDS patient, no interleukin-2

Response of lymphocytes from an AIDS patient, interleukin-2 added

Figure 18. Partial restoration of an AIDS patient's immune function by interleukin-2.

Lymphocytes from AIDS patients perform very poorly in laboratory tests of immune function, but the addition of certain lymphokines to these test systems can improve responsiveness. A lymphokine called interleukin-2 is particularly promising (Fig. 18) and the definite possibility exists that this or other lymphokines could be useful in therapy. It must be stressed, however, that lymphokines would have to be used in combination with anti-HIV drugs such as Zidovudine, since increased T-cell activation induced by lymphokines would be expected to activate latent HIV within T-helper lymphocytes (see p.2 and Fig. 2).

Chapter 8

Other Human Immunodeficiency Viruses

In 1986 a second virus capable of causing AIDS was isolated from 2 men from West Africa, one from Guinea Bissau and the other from Cape Verde Islands. This part of Africa has so far suffered a lower prevalence of HIV infection than Central Africa. The new virus, now named HIV-2, has similar biological properties to HIV-1, i.e., it binds via envelope glycoprotein to the T4 molecule of T-helper lymphocytes and macrophages, can remain latent inside these infected cells and can proliferate rapidly to bring about severe depletion of T4-positive cells and severe immunodeficiency. Preliminary information, however, suggests that HIV-2 may not be quite as pathogenic as HIV-1. HIV-2 has not yet spread extensively in the developed world but has a high prevalence in West Africa.

HIV-2 shows only about 40% similarity with HIV-1 at the gene level, i.e., its nucleotide sequence and the structure of its component proteins are much more different from HIV-1 than the differences seen between various isolates of HIV-1. On the other hand, HIV-2 is much more closely related (approximately 80% similarity) to a virus (simian immunodeficiency virus) which is able to cause an AIDS-like syndrome in some species of monkey. It is now believed that a (probably large) family of viruses exists in monkeys and man, with varying potential to cause immunodeficiency; indeed HIV-3 has reportedly been isolated in recent months.

HIV-2 is sufficiently different from HIV-1 to often escape detection in ELISA tests for HIV-1 antibodies, and specific tests for HIV-2 may be required to screen donated blood for transfusion. It is most earnestly hoped that lessons learnt from extensive studies of HIV-1 will be applicable to prevention and control of infection with HIV-2 and other human immunodeficiency viruses.

Chronology of the AIDS Epidemic

1959	HIV *may* be present in Zaire
1972	HIV present in healthy persons in rural Uganda
1976	First AIDS cases in Central Africa ⎫
1978	First AIDS cases in USA ⎬ diagnosed retrospectively
1980	First AIDS cases in Europe ⎭
1981	AIDS recognized as a new clinical entity
1983	First AIDS cases in Australasia/Asia
1983/84	HIV isolated and major biological properties determined
1985	ELISA for HIV antibodies developed
1986	HIV-2 isolated from West Africa
1987	Zidovudine shown to be clinically useful
1988	HIV-3 isolated
	Education is the only weapon against AIDS
1991	1–2 million AIDS cases and 80–200 million HIV carriers predicted
2000	Probably no HIV vaccine before this date Effective drugs may become available to prevent development of AIDS in HIV carriers

Appendix 2

Some Basic Immunology

AIDS is the consequence of destruction of the immune system by a newly discovered virus, HIV. To understand fully how this comes about it is necessary to appreciate some of the basic workings of the immune system. This extremely complex network of cells and mediators is responsible for:

(1) *Recognizing* any substance that is foreign to the body and which potentially could be a threat to it. Molecules that can stimulate an immune response are called *antigens.*

(2) *Responding* to that antigen to neutralize, destroy and remove it from the body.

(3) Retaining a *memory* of the first encounter with a given antigen so that any subsequent encounter will bring about an accelerated response.

Two types of cells are primarily responsible for these activities – *macrophages* and *lymphocytes.* Macrophages are important in the earliest stages of the immune response, being able to engulf particulate antigens and process them to a form that can be recognized by lymphocytes. These latter cells come in three major types, each with a particular job to do.

B-lymphocytes ('B' refers to the fact that these cells come to maturity in the bone marrow) are responsible for producing proteins called *antibodies*, which have a basic structure of 4 polypeptide chains – 2 identical 'heavy' and 2 identical 'light' chains arranged in the shape of a 'Y' (Fig. 19). Each heavy and light chain has a terminal 'variable' region which defines the shape of a binding site for antigen. Since each molecule of antibody has a unique binding site, it will bind only one antigen. Antigen fits into the binding site like a key into a lock (Fig. 20).

Antibodies are responsible for neutralizing dangerous materials in the body, such as toxins and viruses, and antigens complexed to antibody can be readily taken up and digested by macrophages.

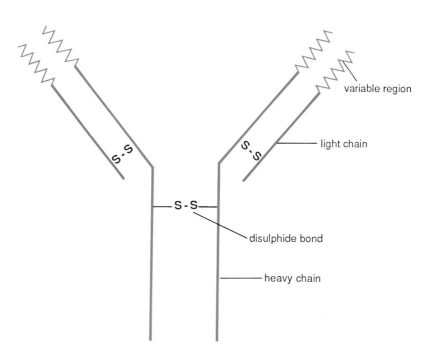

variable region

light chain

disulphide bond

heavy chain

Figure 19.   Basic structure of antibody.

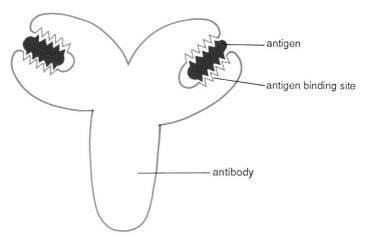

antigen

antigen binding site

antibody

Figure 20.   Binding of antibody to antigen.

B-lymphocytes have antibody molecules on their surfaces which form a *receptor* for antigen. Each B-lymphocyte has a unique receptor and so can recognize only one antigen. Binding of this specific antigen to the receptor is the initial step in 'priming' the B-lymphocyte to produce large quantities of antibody specific to that antigen, but it cannot continue along this pathway until it receives a second signal (see below).

The second major type of lymphocyte is the 'thymus-derived' or *T-lymphocyte,* and these are divided into three sub-classes: *T-helper, T-cytotoxic* and *T-suppressor* lymphocytes. T-lymphocytes, like B-lymphocytes, have surface receptors for recognizing antigen, each cell has a unique receptor capable of recognizing only one antigen. The T-lymphocyte antigen receptor is similar but not identical to antibody.

T-helper lymphocytes interact with antigen on the surface of macrophages, following which they proliferate to form a clone of cells each able to secrete a variety of soluble hormone-like factors called *lymphokines.* These factors induce all classes of lymphocytes (after they have been primed by antigen) to undergo clonal expansion and to perform their designated functions. There are particular factors for inducing B- and T-lymphocytes to proliferate, B-lymphocytes to secrete antibodies, *cytotoxic T-lymphocytes* to kill target cells such as cancer cells and virus-infected cells, and *suppressor T-lymphocytes* to terminate the immune response once the inducing agent has been neutralized. Lymphokines also induce macrophages to become more efficient at engulfing particular matter, killing bacteria and cancer cells, and presenting antigen to T-helper lymphocytes.

The third major type of lymphocyte is the *natural killer (NK) lymphocyte.* Unlike B- and T-lymphocytes these cells do not have antigen-specific receptors, but instead appear to recognize a common molecule (whose nature is not known) on the surface of cancer cells and virus-infected cells. This enables NK-cells to bind to those target cells and kill them. Again, NK-lymphocytes proliferate and perform their designated functions optimally only after being stimulated by lymphokines.

Note the crucial and central roles of macrophages and T-helper lymphocytes in the immune response. It is little wonder that a virus that can infect these two cell types causes total destruction of all arms of the immune system.

Cellular interactions leading to fully activated effector functions are summarized in Fig. 21.

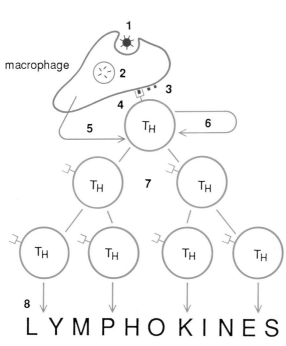

1. Macrophage ingests complex antigen

2. Small antigenic fragments produced

3. These are transferred to the cell surface

4. T-helper lymphocyte recognizes antigen

5. A macrophage product induces...

6. T-helper lymphocyte to secrete lymphokines which ...

7. Induce proliferation

8. Daughter cells secrete large quantities of lymphokines

Lymphokines induce:
– Antigen-primed B-lymphocytes to proliferate and secrete antibodies
– Antigen-primed T-cytotoxic lymphocytes to proliferate and kill target cells
– NK-cells to proliferate and kill target cells
– Macrophages to become more efficient at ingesting, processing and presenting antigen
– Bone marrow progenitor cells to differentiate into mature immune system cells
– Antigen-primed T-suppressor lymphocytes to proliferate and suppress T-helper lymphocyte function, thereby terminating the immune response

Figure 21. Activation of immune effector functions.

Glossary

Acquired immunodeficiency syndrome, AIDS
The late stage of infection with human immunodeficiency virus, when depletion of T-helper lymphocytes has occurred and the body is vulnerable to infections and cancers.

AIDS-related complex, ARC
The stage preceeding AIDS, when constitutional symptoms such as prolonged fever, severe weight loss, diarrhoea, fatigue, night sweats and oral *Candida* infections occur.

Antibody
A protein that is produced as a result of an immunological response to an antigen and which can combine with that antigen.

Antigen
A substance that can induce a detectable immune response when introduced into the body.

Antigenic drift
Subtle changes in the antigenic structure of a micro-organism during the course of an infection which allow it to escape from the immune response.

Anti-idiotype
Antibody directed against the variable region (often the antigen binding site) of an antibody.

Art
One of the genes of HIV responsible for pathogenesis – anti-repressor of transactivation.

Attenuated
Rendered less virulent.

Autoimmunity
Immunological reactivity against self.

Azidothymidine (AZT)
(See Zidovudine).

B-lymphocyte
Cell type responsible, after activation, for producing antibodies.

Bone marrow transplantation
Injection of immune system progenitor cells into an immunologically deficient patient .

Carrier (eg., of HIV)
Infected person showing no symptoms of disease, but able to infect others.

Core
Internal structure of a virus.

Cytotoxic T-lymphocyte
Cell type capable of killing virus-infected and cancer cells.

Deletion mutant
Pathogen which has been attenuated by removal of certain genes responsible for virulence.

Dementia
Deteriorated mental state.

Deoxyribonucleic acid (DNA)
The chemical carrier of genetic information.

Dideoxycytidine
A drug which inhibits HIV proliferation and is being used in experimental therapy of AIDS.

Eczema
Scabs, scales or crusts of the skin.

ELISA
Enzyme-linked immunosorbent assay – a sensitive technique for measuring levels of antibodies or antigens in body fluids.

Encephalitis
Inflammation of the brain.

Env
The gene which codes for the envelope proteins of HIV.

Envelope
The outer structure of a virus.

Escherichia coli
A bacillus which inhabits the colon.

Factor VIII
A factor required for blood clotting. Haemophiliacs are deficient in this factor.

Gag
The gene which codes for the core proteins of HIV.

Gene
A segment of DNA which codes for a protein.

Genome
The entire complement of genes of an organism.

Giant cell
Multinucleated cell formed by fusion of several individual cells.

Glycoprotein
A compound consisting of protein and carbohydrate.

gp41
The transmembrane component of the HIV envelope glycoprotein, molecular weight 41,000 daltons.

gp120
The external component of the HIV envelope glycoprotein, molecular weight 120,000 daltons.

Haemophilia
A blood clotting disorder.

Helper T-lymphocyte
A type of lymphocytes which co-operates with other lymphocyte types in the performance of their designated immunological functions.

Human immunodeficiency virus (HIV)
The causative agent of AIDS and related disorders.

Idiotype
The antigen-binding part of an antibody molecule or T-cell receptor, or a site close to it.

Immunofluorescence test
A technique for detecting antigens or antibodies in which an antibody against the substance to be detected is tagged with a chemical that fluoresces when examined using an ultraviolet microscope.

Immunogenicity
Ability of a substance to induce a detectable immune response.

Immunological activation
Conversion of resting immune system cells into an active state capable of performing effector functions.

Interferons
Proteins produced by virus-infected cells which protect other cells against infection.

Interleukin-2
A lymphokine with many different activities, including the stimulation of clonal proliferation of activated lymphocytes.

Kaposi's sarcoma
A relatively benign tumour of the skin which can, however, become aggressive and spread to the internal organs of immunocompromised patients such as those with AIDS.

Killer cells
Cytotoxic T-lymphocytes or natural killer lymphocytes.

Latency period
The time between infection and appearance of symptoms.

Latent infection
An infection with no visible symptoms.

Lymphadenopathy
Swollen lymph glands.

Lymphocyte
White blood cell able to specifically recognize and respond to antigens.

Lymphokines
Soluble hormone-like products of activated lymphocytes with diverse effects on immune system cells and other cell types.

Lymphoma
A tumour of the lymphoid system.

Macrophage
White blood cell capable of engulfing, processing and presenting antigen to lymphocytes.

Monokines
Soluble hormone-like products of macrophages with diverse effects on immune system cells and other cell types.

Natural killer (NK-) cells
A type of lymphocyte distinct from B- and T-lymphocytes which can attack virus-infected and cancer cells without prior sensitization.

Neutralizing antibody
Antibody capable of preventing the infection of target cells by viruses.

Neutropenia
Abnormally low number of neutrophils in the blood.

Neutrophils
Scavenger white blood cells which stain easily with neutral dyes.

Nonoxynol-9
A spermicidal agent which also inactivates HIV.

Nucleotide
The structural unit of DNA and RNA, comprising a purine (adenine or guanine) or pyrimidine (thymine, cytosine or uracil) base, phosphoric acid and a sugar (ribose in RNA, deoxyribose in DNA). The sequence of nucleotides within a gene determines the amino acid sequence of the protein product of the gene.

Opportunistic infection
Infection by a normally non-infectious or non-pathogenic organism at a time when the immune system is defective.

3' ORF
An HIV gene (3' open reading frame) whose protein product appears to be required for the establishment of a latent infection.

p18 and p24
Major HIV core proteins with molecular weights of 18,000 and 24,000 daltons.

Peptide T
A synthetic peptide which competitively inhibits binding of HIV to T4-positive cells.

Placebo
An inactive substance given to the control group in a clinical trial.

Pneumocystis carinii
A fungus responsible for the most common opportunistic infection in AIDS patients, *P. carinii* pneumonia.

Pol
The gene which codes for HIV's reverse transcriptase.

Polymorphs
Scavenger white blood cells with multi-lobed nuclei.

Polypeptide
A compound of several amino acids.

Progenitor cells
Cells from which other cells are derived.

Radioimmune precipitation
A sensitive technique for detecting antibodies against HIV, which measures precipitation of radioactively-labelled HIV proteins.

Receptor
A molecule on a cell surface with specific affinity for a particular agent.

Recombinant DNA technology
The insertion of an isolated gene into the genome of another organism (often the bacillus E. coli) so that the latter can be cultured and large quantities of the protein product of the inserted gene obtained from the culture supernatant.

Retrovirus
A group of viruses whose genetic code is made up of RNA and which possess an enzyme, reverse transcriptase, which converts RNA to DNA. The latter can be incorporated into the host cell genome.

Reverse transcriptase
An enzyme which converts RNA into DNA. This is the reverse of normal transcription (DNA → RNA → protein).

Ribonucleic acid (RNA)
Messenger RNA, transfer RNA and ribosomal RNA are involved in converting the DNA genetic message into proteins. In certain viruses, RNA rather than DNA forms the genetic code.

Simian immunodeficiency viruses (SIV)
A group of viruses which infect various species of monkey and which may cause an AIDS-like syndrome.

Slim disease
African name for AIDS, so called because of the extreme loss of weight seen in its victims.

Soluble T4
A recombinant DNA-derived form of T4 (the HIV receptor) which inhibits binding of the virus to cell-associated T4. An experimental therapy for AIDS.

Sor
Short open reading frame — an HIV gene whose protein product is important for penetration into the target cell.

Suppressor T-lymphocyte
Cell type responsible for regulating the immune response and terminating it after successful removal of antigen.

T4 (modern term CD4)
Molecule present at high density on the surface of T-helper lymphocytes and at low density on some macrophages. The cellular receptor for HIV.

Tat
Transactivator of transcription, an HIV gene involved in pathogenesis. Its product enhances the rate of transcription of other viral genes, thereby increasing the rate of proliferation.

T-lymphocyte
Type of lymphocyte that matures in the thymus. In contrast to B-lymphocytes, they do not produce antibodies. Divided into 3 classes: T-helper, T-cytotoxic and T-suppressor.

Transcription
The conversion of a DNA nucleotide sequence into the corresponding messenger RNA sequence.

Translation
The conversion of a messenger RNA sequence into the corresponding amino acid sequence of a protein.

Western blot
A highly specific test for detecting antibodies to HIV, used to confirm a positive ELISA test .

Zidovudine
Also known as Azidothymidine. The only drug discovered so far to have proven therapeutic benefits in AIDS patients. It inhibits HIV proliferation by becoming incorporated into the growing DNA chain in place of thymidine, thereby inhibiting reverse transcription.

FESTIVAL

A Collective Tribute
to the Art of Celebration

Published by Proost

Thanks for buying this book.

It's been created to be a tribute to the art of celebrating and to explore all the benefits celebration has to us as human beings.

However, proceeds from the book will also go towards supporting the wellbeing and mental health of everyday people, particularly at UK Festivals.

For more info visit **spacetobreathe.eu**

TABLE OF CONTENTS

INTRODUCTION

'A Tribute to the Art of Celebration' by Andy Freeman

Welcome to 'Festival.'

This book has been a little while in the making and begins with an absurd story. Last Summer I was at the Greenbelt Festival at Boughton House near Kettering. Greenbelt is a joyous festival, set in a lush green environment and one that mixes art and spirituality – two things that make me tick. Understandably I like being there.

But Greenbelt 2018 was different for me as our little wellbeing company called Space to Breathe had been invited to run a venue and some programming. This was an exciting development but meant a stressful and busy lead-up the festival itself.

By the middle Saturday of Greenbelt, I was exhausted. Things had gone well and the tiredness and stress wasn't a problem or failure – however I knew I needed to face up to how I felt or find a way to recharge as we had two more busy days in front of us.

Usually, when I reach a place of extreme tiredness – rest and an early night are always part of the solution. Although our wellbeing is often complex, sometimes simple questions around my sleep, my diet or exercise can be illuminating. But here at Greenbelt, as a light sleeper at the best of times an evening of sleeping on the floor in a damp tent didn't feel appealing.

I clocked off at 8pm and my daughter Lucy asked me whether I'd like to go and see a band. With the thought of that damp roll-mat in my mind I said yes very quickly. It ended up being a very wise decision.

For the next few hours, and with We Are Scientists and Carny Villains as the soundtrack, I danced and moshed out all my stress. Being 50 years old, my dancing probably isn't pretty and is unskilled but I can assure you, I had fun. I even broke my little toe – now a permanent memento to a novel way of enhancing wellbeing.

The next morning, I pondered the night before. There was something counter-intuitive about dancing to rest and yet it had worked. I felt alive again, my anxiety had disappeared and I felt happy and content. Given that I had jumped around like a mad thing for a few hours how did I feel restored?

When I returned home, I sat my coach and friend Holly Crosby (who's contributed to this book) and asked how could this be? We laughed as I retold the story but Holly's wisdom was this – fun gave me strength and gave me life. Holly asked me to have a look through my daily life and the things I spent time on. How much time did I give to fun? The answer was not very much.

This Greenbelt experience opened my eyes. We spend so much time speaking out wellbeing in a preventative sense. It's estimated 1 in 4 of us will face some sort of mental health challenge each year[1]. Many initiatives and groups have sprung up to support this growing challenge – and rightly so. So many professions are now citing stress, depression and anxiety as key factors in resignations or long term ill-health. For example, a National Education Union poll in 2018 found that 26% of UK teachers with less than five years of teaching experience planned to quit by 2024[2]. This must change.

However, if we only discuss the negative challenges of wellbeing we only see half the story. We all have mental health and our flourishing is equally important as the prevention of mental health problems. We have the chance to thrive. I had become adept at addressing areas of concern (stress/anxiety) but had seemingly ignored something which enabled me to flourish – having fun.

This journey brought me to Festivals and to this book.

Over the past year I've met many people who have struggled with their mental health at Festivals. The highs of the crowd and the event can also lead to paralyzing lows of stress and depression. We've worked hard over the past months to address these issues and we were thrilled to create a 'Wellbeing Guide' for people attending 2019's Tramlines Festival in Sheffield[3].

But this book represents another side of the coin. Festival is about growing our wellbeing through flourishing and particularly through the art of celebration. It is a tribute to joy and thankfulness.

Represented in these pages are articles and ideas from other members of the Space to Breathe team – Ben, Nicky and myself.

We are also thrilled to have guest contributions from others and they express the varied nature of celebration.

Richard Passmore shares a beautiful and prosaic ode to celebration in all its forms – relationships, snow-days, childbirth and indeed festivals – the amazing nature of tears and the communal nature of joy.

Martin Daws simple 'Thank you Card' traces back the origins of sharing a greeting card. Celebration can be messy – it is rarely pure happiness and often includes sorrow or questions.

Grenfell Singing is a beautiful example of that idea. The horror of the Grenfell Fire in 2017 will remain with many of us forever. Yet the applause given to firefighters shows that even there we can celebrate someone.

British Record Skipping Champion, Beth Rookwood and Holly Crosby both touch on the idea of celebrating success. This is something we hear time and again it classrooms or boardrooms and to be honest, maybe we're not that good at it. Sometimes it's time to cheer and celebrate. Beth does this with Prosecco and a willingness to say 'Yay!' Holly encourage us to see the things we're good at and accept them.

Poetry from Talitha Fraser and Helen Dean develop this idea. Celebration has a role and it is good for you. "Get Party Poppers" is one of Talitha's pieces of wisdom.

Beth Keith shares the moving story of her daughter's journey to learning and expressing dance. We can 'dance it out' even in moments of difficulty as well as in joy.

Lucie Shuker beautifully the concept of embracing festival and celebration as a gift and the unique sense of community it brings.

These contributions lead us to a wonderful and freeing piece of wisdom. Festivals are good for us. These parties for the masses give us an opportunity to be ourselves, the concept this book concludes with.

My friend Jonny Baker issued me with a wonderful challenge one day. He said my role was to be "a little bit more Andy Freeman every day." This has stuck with me.

I have so many roles – father, husband, director, citizen, friend, godparent, grandfather, sponsor, mentor or supporter. Each one of these roles is vital and wonderful. But the thing I'm to do each day is to be a little bit more myself.

I don't have to be the Andy that does this, or the Andy that these people see. I'm to be me, plain and simple. And I've found Andy likes to have fun, and that it is good for him.

Festivals give us so many opportunities to celebrate, to be ourselves and to express joy. The contributors in this book give credit for that but also give us the tools to celebrate each day. Celebration can be a wonderful tool to aid our wellbeing and it is deeply accessible.

I enjoyed writing the poem 'Drum-Thud Misfit' for this book as I remembered my times attending a moshy and muddy Reading Festival in the 80's. I remember feeling a sense of belonging when so often I felt isolated. I hated leaving each year, wishing a place like this existed at home. Festivals can be those once in a moment times of happiness and joy but so many of the principles of celebration can be accessed always in our lives and in simple ways. Celebration doesn't have to be a one-off but can become a rhythm, a way of life.

I hope you enjoy the book.

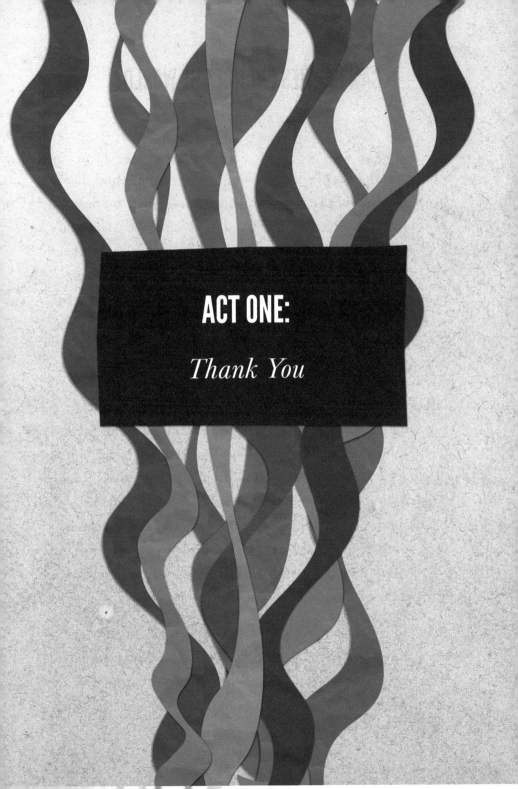

ACT ONE:

Thank You

CAN PARTIES CHANGE THE WORLD?

by Richard Passmore

Out beyond ideas of right or wrong there's a party and there's people sitting on the stairs, shoulder to shoulder putting the world in perspective and in doing so processing the chaos that's always swirling around them. You will also find us in the kitchen, whilst the music plays and the heat rises with the dancers in front room, over a beer by the worktop the alliance of strangers, where camaraderie is formed and the soul is fed, through ideas, presence and random connections.

A love is celebrated in a hotel, a moment where this place of business becomes sacred. Where once finished the legal and robotic matrimonial agents of state, give way to something far older, far more ancient, shaped by but reaching back beyond ideas of organised religion. A friend in priestly orders takes his long embroidered stole, and wraps the couple's hands together, our hands, and whilst words are said few are needed. Later instead of the disco or dance, stories are told by guests, stories not of the couple, but of the lives of those sharing the day, and there are stories that stick and stay once the day is over.

A home is being made, our home, walls knocked through to make a place of welcome. Large enough to build a bigger table. The builders are gone and small community, no a small army of friends move in, armed with paint brushes and rollers. Music

12

plays into the night, and the workers break roughly tare pizza into pieces because they never cut it properly at the takeaway and the cutlery is yet to be found. This bread is broken and beers are passed around, the symbolism lost for many, but not by the recipients of the generous gift of time from friends. The work party is simply that - a party, a festival of life, sitting on paint tins and boxes, listening to a small radio, rather than in a field on blankets with a booming sound system. But like that larger festival, many will pass through this room in the years to come as it transformed into a well-used and welcoming space. A web of relationships will be formed from here that reach across generational boundaries, into skate parks and homes and out to those on the edge.

In the garden, on a warm spring day new life is recognised. Notes are placed in a box that won't be opened by this child for at least a decade and is still yet to be opened, that's a celebration yet to be planned. Wisdom and prayers drawn from the community gathered in the green space, written on slips and placed inside this now sacred box. Once again the friend in religious orders reaches back beyond recent history, and touches the child's forehead with that same embroidered stole.

In this year of the Golden Pig, and the mothers who carried children for many months now place them together on the sofa to celebrate the end of this first year of life. To forget for a moment the sleep deprived nights, and the days that draw slowly. Strangers drawn together in a class for novices, still in touch many months later, share the expertise they have gained and who they are becoming. Streams merge as family wisdom passed down the generations is generously shared to this wider family, some of it will simply be forgotten but much will be added to the flow of life.

The clans are gathering. Those with open houses back in their towns and cities and networked together through a shared love of community, descend on this temporary festival field. A space dedicated for 48 hours to this network of activists, dreamers, schemers and friends. Tents are pitched, bottles are opened, spaces are saved for late comers and the community swells with friends of friends of friends. The growth is always at the edge, as newcomers are welcomed and new stories heard and absorbed. New ways of connecting are discussed, simple acts of service both here and to take back to their local communities are discovered. As the evening draws in, sat around the open fire, a symbol so ancient many sense they are part of a greater story, and whilst the narrative of the resurrection remains unsaid it does not go unheard.

The town wakes to a covering of white. Children search the web for news that school might be cancelled and cheers go up from across the breakfast tables as they find out. Calls are made and plans are hatched, sledges, trays, bags and even surf boards are dusted off as we head for the hills. The temporary community formed on this snow day might not be seen again for many years or more, but for now there's a party on the slope where everyone is welcome.

It's time for another temporary community, but this now happens every year. The first was to the celebrate the newly opened skate park and green after years of fundraising by a bunch of teenagers who all but a few had written off. Now with its music, stalls, competitions, something new has emerged, it permanence lasting beyond the day it takes place. And somehow like fetes of old the whole of community gather to celebrate each year, to party, to barbecue and be reminded by young people what a small group of committed individuals can achieve.

It is time to move, no matter how painful it is to break the embedded ties into this now much extended community, to this house, no longer covered by that army of painters, but formed by the tears and laughter of nearly a decade of relationships and celebrations. Another party is planned, perhaps a final farewell. Stuff collected over the last ten years is shared around, a young couple setting up homes welcome a table and chairs that they have sat on since their teens, other items are packed and many are sold to pay for the party at the local curry house that has become home from home for many in the extensive web of relationships that have been formed. Old friends are present, and young people who have shared the journey now gather as friends, some with children of their own, different strands of the web are sat together and a table far longer that could ever be included in the house that was our home is laden with food.

As the lunch draws to an end and we look back on the years in this place we are reminded how much we have been supported and nourished by the celebrations we have attended. How often during these times of great celebration that it was not only tears of joy that have been shed? How we have sat on steps away from the noise and the bustle, at times with and without words. How the world for many was crumbling whilst the celebrations went on inside, and how somehow that discongruity created a space for the fullness of our humanity to meet. So, our parting words to the gathered congregation are of thankfulness and a reminder that parties are far more important than meetings.

GRATITUDE

by Andy Freeman

The simple practice of gratitude can be life changing.

In 2018, as part of the work of Dr.Fuschia Sirois, a gratitude wall was erected in my home city of Sheffield. The project was striking and thought-provoking but was backed by more than what the Guardian once called the "Oprah bandwagon" of positive wellbeing.[4]

Multiple studies have shown that a positive approach to gratitude and thankfulness helps with stress and depression, sorts out relationships, aids sleep and builds wellbeing and resilience (e.g. Sirois/Wood 2017.[5])

Studies have also shown simple gratitude tools like making a daily list have positive effects on wellbeing in similar areas (e.g. Wood/Froh/Geraghty 2010.[6])

In a book that recognises the value of celebration, gratitude is a central issue. We find it a lot harder to be grateful than you'd think.

The phrase 'thank you' is a common one in UK culture. On the whole, in our manners-based culture we are OK at saying thanks when its needed. However, we are also pretty good at what Kate Fox called 'Eeyoreness'[7] – we see the negative whether it be the weather, the likelihood of sporting defeat or our ability to mess up.

When it comes to gratitude, we can find this hard and a sense of being hard-done-by can grow. When this is added to difficult times in life, the simple question on gratitude may be 'why bother?'

Here I've found the wisdom of spirituality a vast ocean of wisdom. Spiritual traditions often do gratitude well – they foster a sense of thankfulness.

"Wear gratitude like a cloak and it will feed every corner of your life"

–Rumi[8]

Rumi has stumbled across a profound truth. If we begin to be grateful, it changes our attitude and in doing so changes all of our selves.

When I'm struggling and feel like life is being unkind to me, I'll naturally put up defences. This is one of our basic human mechanisms – when we are in danger, we circle the wagons.

Gratitude has the opposite effect. It removes some of the hostility from the world around us. It makes us open; it gives us the potential to be vulnerable and trusting with others. It says good can happen here.

"Today, let us swim wildly and joyously in gratitude"

"Gratitude is wine for the soul. Go on. Get drunk"

–Rumi[9]

I love both of those quotes. Gratitude is a lavish and fulsome thing.

Think about it. When we are grateful, we will smile. It warms us. It's very hard to be truly grateful and at the same time be truly grumpy. I think this is because gratefulness comes from deep within us. It's something of the soul (see Act Four for more.)

The more we have of being grateful the more it gives to us. It is a wide source.

A while ago I first practiced the principle of writing down ten things I was grateful for each morning. Some days this flowed easily. When things are good, ten is a short list. However, following hard days this list writing took time. I'd be forced to be thankful for the milkman or for the air I breathe.

But here's the weird thing. It was those days when this practice changed me. Why shouldn't I be thankful for milk? A year later a short stomach illness resulted in me not being able to eat or drink any dairy products. Then I realised what a gift the taste of cheese or butter was. Everything can be good and glorious – why not be thankful?

Poet Maya Angelou once wrote "let gratitude be the pillow upon which you kneel to say your nightly prayer.[10]" We are in a world deserving of our gratefulness.

So many good things come into our lives and often by accident. Have you noticed how often we make plans; we work in a way to see certain results and yet often the best things come completely without explanation or warning?

What do we do with a world like that?

Gratefulness at least allows us to say there are things that happen in our world to which we owe gratitude to others or to a sense of the other that can only be expressed in a thankful attitude. Maybe this is why spirituality does indeed do gratefulness so well.

"If the only prayer you said was thank
you, that would be enough"

–Meister Eckhart[11]

THE SIMPLE THANK YOU CARD
WRITTEN WITH THANKS

by Martin Daws

Thank the tree that the card is made from - thank the rain on the tree - thank the clouds that drop the rain - thank the mountains that the clouds form on - thank the glaciers that cut the mountains that the clouds form on - thank the sea the water in the clouds comes from - thank the sun that warms the water in the sea - thank the air that forms the wind that moves the clouds - thank the earth.

Breathe.

Thank the foresters that cut the tree - thank the forester's NGO for planting the forest - thank the environment that was destroyed by the forest - thank the chain saw makers - the steel manufacturers - the lorry drivers - the vehicle manufacturers - the seafarers - ship builders - crane operators - the trainers of crane operators - the makers of cranes - the producers of design and presentation software used by the makers of cranes - thank the makers of the designer's and producer's computer hardware - thank the paper mill workers - the paper mill architects - the owners of the paper mill.

Breathe.

Thank the oil industry engineers - the oil rig roughnecks - the oil company

employees and executives - thank the oil - thank the millions of years that compounded the life of the place where the tree grew deep enough underground to cathargise its carbon into oil - thank the carbon - thank the tree before the tree the forester cut down - thank the forester before the forester that cut the tree and thank the forester before the forester that cut the tree before the tree that the forester cut down and thank the forester's parents grandparents family friends lovers teachers acquaintances ancestors.

Breathe.

Thank the plastic factory workers - the cellophane scientists - the product price algorithm analysts - the retail assistants - the bank workers - the economists - the politicians - the business people and the people who write the messages. Breathe. Thank all their family friend's lovers' teachers' acquaintances ancestors.

Breathe.

Thank all of the above - all of the below - all of the forgotten - all of the anonymous and unknown - all of the too distant for concern - the too uncomfortable to hold - the too infinite to touch - the impossible ocean of us - every ever and ever of life.

Breathe.

Thank the person you bought the simple thank you card to thank.

GRENFELL SINGING

An anonymous reflection

On 14th June 2017, fire engulfed Grenfell Tower in West London, killing 71 people and leaving countless others with unthinkable trauma, without homes of their own and a community deep with scars.

For so many of us that lived around the tower, life has changed. I was woken in the night by shouts and screams and stepped out into the street to look up at the burning building. I'm not sure I looked down again for hours.

The next day and for hundreds of days after that, all we saw was the charred and burnt out wreck of Grenfell Tower. It became a symbol of pain, and of anger. It was the first view of each of our monthly silent marches to remember those who died.

Nowadays it's covered in plastic with a green heart at the top. A gesture I guess but to be honest, all I see is a burnt-out tomb. I knew people there. How could I feel anything else?

When you feel this amount of pain, simple things feel stupid.

I remember the first time I heard someone laugh after the fire. It felt insulting, arrogant. How can they laugh? It was an injustice. Surely all laughter now is inappropriate.

I know that will sound silly to you, but that's how I felt. Pain left little space for anyone else's world. Of course, these were laughs from those who'd not felt my scars. If I thought about it, the TV still had comedy shows. Music still played. Goals were still scored. But for me, it felt a world away.

On the Sunday after the fire, a local church held a morning service outside on the road under the Westway. There was a band playing and lots of people – I remember that. We were very blessed that so many people had journeyed to Grenfell to offer help, to volunteer. I was so proud of the faith groups for the way they helped. It felt right to be there, but I stood near the back and occasionally sat on the pavements edge. I didn't want to engage too much.

Towards the end of the service (remember we're on the street) a group of Fire Engine's came along and needed to get through. Immediately the singing stopped and everyone got hold of the chairs and stuff and moved them so they could get through.

At that time, hundreds of firefighters were still at the Tower, searching the wreckage and making the building safe. They all looked exhausted.

As they drove past someone started clapping. Then others. Soon everyone was applauding as these three Fire Engines slowly drove past us. The people inside them cried and waved. It was beautiful.

I clapped hard. I remember my hands began to hurt.

Then I felt tears and for the first time since the fire, they weren't painful tears. They were proud. They spoke joy.

As the chairs were replaced the band started singing a hymn. I tried to remember for this piece what the song was, but I can't. What I do remember though is I felt deep deep emotion. I sang hard. I sang till my throat hurt. It meant something.

Andy told me he was writing some things about celebration and asked if I'd write something too. We had met that weekend as he was a volunteer who'd come to help. We stayed in touch and he asked me to write about that Sunday, those Fire Engines, that applause and that singing.

Celebrating something isn't always happy or fun. Even now, two years on and with the fight for justice still unresolved, the memory of that night is too much for me. But in those following days I did find things to celebrate and be grateful for.

I'm grateful for those firemen and firewomen.

I'm grateful for my neighbours and friends and for the deeper friendships we have now.

I'm grateful for the lives of those who were lost and for the lives of those who made it through.

I'm grateful to have a place to live and that I can share it.

I'm grateful for fresh air, for friends and family.

I can go on.

Life is painful. It hurts often.

I don't know why that is or what that means.

But I do know that celebrating those brave men and women that day helped me.

Thanks for reading.

MEDITATION

Grateful Tree

This meditation needs a small tree, plant or bush – something with branches strong enough to tie someone on.

It also needs some luggage tags and a pen.

Gratefulness is such a valuable and helpful practice.

This meditation is about taking one month and coming up with three things to be grateful for every day.

1. Each day, take three luggage tags and finish this sentence. 'I am grateful for ...'

2. Take each tag and tie it to your plant or tree.

3. Repeat this for one month. Make sure you do three each day, even if you don't feel like it.

4. After one month, you'll have a tree full of tags. Reflect on them. Life can feel hard but even the simplest of things can bring joy and show us we have things to be thankful for.

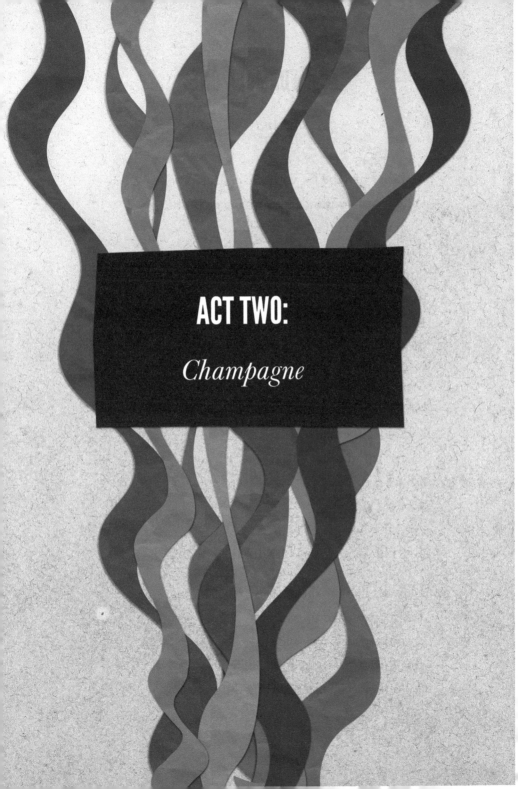

ACT TWO:

Champagne

FORMULA ONE

by Andy Freeman

I always like the bit with the champagne.
There are hundreds of ways to celebrate,
Speeches go on wax and wane.
High fives and celebration,
Smiling winners, losers pain,
Punching fists
And songs refrain
But I always like the bit with the champagne.

I always like the bit with the champagne.
Shake the bottle
Cliquot's the name.
It's a rich man's way
Of joy and pain.
Copse, Maggots
And the Brands Chicane.
But I always like the bit with the champagne.

I always like the bit with the champagne.
I don't even like the stuff
And the excess is a shame.
But I like they make a fuss of achieving
That they celebrate winning the game.

I like the overalls, the teams,

The mechanics are all the same.

And I always like the bit with the champagne.

CELEBRATION'S WHAT YOU NEED!

Celebration as a rhythm of life

by Beth Rookwood

I'm of the Record Breakers generation – a prime time kids TV show– where super-energetic, massively enthusiastic, impressively non-fashionista hosts tracked the nail-biting attempts of people across the world seeking a place in the Guinness Book of Records.

Their theme song sung by the irrepressible Roy Castle, (see You-Tube if bells are not immediately ringing) contained many repeats of the phrase: 'Dedication's what you need.... if you wanna be a Record Breaker...Yeah!'

Now, as a Record Breaker* myself I can vouch for the truth in the lyric; hours of practice, early morning training, competitions, parents as taxi drivers etc.; dedication was certainly needed to get my team to that high point where we received the highly prized blue and red t-shirts with the RB logo on. All that <u>hard work had</u> finally paid off – the 'work till you drop then

* My British Record attempt was in Skipping. The record we went for was the highest number of people in a rope doing the most number of skips. Surprisingly difficult. I think 100 of us from skipping clubs all over the country managed 13 skips...was it worth the trip from the Midlands to a workshop in a deserted part of North London? Absolutely!

work till it's done' approach to life, one step further entrenched in my teenage self.

Of course, the challenge to that approach comes when, outside of the 'record breaking regime,' a whole way of life appears that still requires a huge amount of dedication but no winning t-shirt: taking exams, filling in job applications, buying a house, writing a novel, developing a project, strengthening a relationship - even just getting the day to day of eat, work, sleep, family, friends done - and the list goes on.

As individuals and as a society, we are good at the dedication thing; we know long hours, constant communication, missed days off, email-checking on holidays, hiking up our gym/ weight/ strength targets. We know the grueling grind of making something happen – but without records, our dedication rarely has a satisfactory end point, and we know this too – it's exhausting! We know that never-ending mountain to climb, the burn out, the sense of feeling trapped by a goal where the posts continue to move further away.

Even with records, the British Record pales in comparison to the Global (it's ok, I learned to live with it), the person that breaks the record becomes the new nemesis, circumstances may change which require a new approach: dedication without records is relentless, and on its own can break us.

So how to break this 'dedication's what you need' culture? How to stop the burn out, exhaustion, disappointment, disillusion?

For me: Prosecco.

Not in a hide-away-and-drown-it-all-away-in-a-pretty-glass kind of way (though if that dark hole looms replace 'prosecco' with something else that makes you happy; hot chocolate works nearly as well for me), but in a 'let's celebrate' kind of way. Is there any other noise that consistently produces a 'yaaaaay' like the pop of a cork?

This sound is the sound now heard in my kitchen most Friday nights. Throughout the week the bubbles sit in the fridge door. I see the bottle, and it reminds me to notice things to celebrate; things that, as the 'pop' goes on Friday, are spoken out and heard by whoever else is in the room; people who are invited to raise their glass and share their own moments of celebration too, however small, however non-global, however much they will remain unnoticed by the world around them.

For me, finding a weekly rhythm of celebration punctuates the daily and life-long dedication with fun, hope, gratitude, the sense of a pursuit well done, and even rest as I allow myself to smile and reflect on what has been; the journey which is now as precious as the goal. It allows for a noticing of the many wins, to acknowledge records broken in my own life, as I achieve new things, face and overcome my fears, see progress, recognize growth and celebrate it all! For why shouldn't we? And why wouldn't we – why only wait until that end point to celebrate, a point which might move away from us at any moment??

So yes, dedication is what we need…but I am finding that celebration is essential for the dedication to remain life-giving rather than life-sucking, a pursuit I continue to choose, rather than a long slog I feel trapped by.

And, hello? An extra reason to pop a cork and raise a glass on a Friday night? Count me in!

CELEBRATING SUCCESS

by Holly Crosby

I'm going to be talking about 'success' a lot here, so let me set the scene.

Not too long ago a very rude (you can probably tell where this is going) man barked at me 'are you a success' before deciding if I could speak at one of his events. Turns out, from that sole phone call, I didn't actually want to speak at one of his events! Was I his definition of a success - absolutely not. Am I mine – yes!

We're all individual; our experiences, our makeup, our world all help to shape us and how we define success. In which case, it makes no sense to compare ourselves or celebrate or successes based on someone else's opinion.

Now that's cleared up, I want you to think back to the last time you achieved something. It could be big; it could be small. But whatever it is it's unique to you. Now my question is 'did you celebrate it?' Because we often don't. We often let our successes drift by without even acknowledging them. Why? Probably the number one reason is that we don't want to look like a 'show off'. In fact, we're probably more likely to play it down rather than shout about it!

Yet if a friend shared a success of theirs, we'd probably congratulate them rather than think of them as showing off. We're often far kinder to others than ourselves.

Celebrating our successes has so many benefits…

- ✓ It motivates us to keep going and to do even more!
- ✓ It makes us feel good
- ✓ We recognise what's worked and can build on it

Start by acknowledging the good that you are doing. And when someone else compliments you, instead of batting it back, simply say 'thank you.' By starting to acknowledge and accept the good, we'll be able to celebrate the success!

What is a 'celebration of success'…

- ✓ It's what you want it to be in that moment! Just as our achievements are unique to us, so should our celebrations.
- ✓ If other's have been a part of it or supported you, share it with them.
- ✓ Keep a record of them. Imagine what a great read that would be!

You've nothing to lose by thinking about what success means to you and how you can celebrate it!

TEN TIPS FOR FEELING WELL AND STAYING WELL

by Nicky Redsell

Being well and maintaining wellbeing is becoming very high profile. One of the reasons for this profile is the fast-paced nature of our world.

> *"The world isn't fast-paced, it's frenetic. People have to be managers of themselves. Time has been managing itself for 15 billion years; we have to manage ourselves in the context of time."*
>
> *–Tony Buzan*[12]

In all our busyness it's as important for us to work out how to sustain ourselves to keep well. Here are 10 top tips to help you maintain your energy levels, motivation and health.

Do not tackle them all at once; instead take small steps in the areas that you feel will most benefit you. Starting small is easier to sustain, especially if you find a specific time for whatever you decide to do. Having a set time will help you, as will putting a tick on a monthly chart each day you achieve your goal. Forming a habit takes time and keeping a record will help.

While the tips are numbered, this does not denote a hierarchy. Select ones that strike you as helpful. You can always try others subsequently.

1: STAY HYDRATED

A staggering 60% of your body consists of water. It is not surprising that staying hydrated is very important as it helps to replace the water you lose during the day. The National Health Service's Eatwell Guide[13] recommends 6–8 glasses of fluid per day, with water being the main percentage of this. It is essential to pay attention to your body, drinking when you feel thirsty. This can be tricky, so try keeping a bottle of water to hand to sip from while working. Take advantage of breaks and do not skip a drink.

2: BE ACTIVE

Not everyone loves getting up early to hit the gym before work (or are able to). While maintaining flexibility and strength benefits our health and emotional wellbeing, fitting exercise in can be a challenge. Exercising with others is a great way to feel encouraged and stay motivated. A walk with a family member, friend or colleague is good, as is going to a fitness class with someone if that appeals. Whatever you decide to try, it is important to do what is manageable and to work with your body's capabilities. You can always build on this subsequently.

3: NURTURE FRIENDSHIPS

Who are the people that accept you warts and all? Whose advice do you trust, and who are you confident is for you? These are the people to keep in contact with, even if this might not be easy to do, especially if they are not local, work full-time or are busy for other reasons. We sometimes substitute face-to-face conversations with social media versions. While this can help to maintain relationships, there is something immensely restorative about spending time with those we hold most dear and letting conversation flow. Set aside a small amount of time to give someone a call or catch up with them over a cup of coffee (or glass of water to keep your hydration levels up).

4: BE MINDFUL

Mindfulness is often described as paying attention to the present moment, and by this we create space for ourselves. By being aware in this way, we can increase our understanding of how we respond to different experiences and people. It can also help us to enjoy the world more fully. All these facets of mindfulness will help to increase our mental resilience and wellbeing.

Here's a method for you to try:

Find a comfortable sitting position. Take a deep breath to loosen any tension in your body. Focus on your breathing, enjoying its rhythm. If you notice your mind wandering, simply allow it to come back to the present moment and resist the temptation to judge yourself. Continue in this manner for 2–3 minutes, increasing the duration over time.[14]

With experience, you might find that you are more able to be mindful in your approach to situations without needing to follow the breathing technique in that moment.

5: BE CURIOUS/TAKE NOTE

Being present in and savouring the moment can help to reaffirm one's life priorities. As we increase our self-awareness, we are more able to make positive choices based on our values. This heightens our sense of connection with others. Take a moment to enjoy the environment you are in. Clear your mind with a few deep breaths and reconnect with yourself. Consider how those alongside you might be feeling. You might want to discuss how your respective days are going. Start a curiosity journal, jotting down new or interesting things that catch your attention during the day. It is interesting to read through your jottings and sketches as your journal grows.

6: KEEP LEARNING AND CREATING

Learning something can be energising and dynamic. It takes us into a new space and our experience broadens. There is evidence that setting learning goals has a positive impact on our wellbeing. Similarly, creating something can give us a sense of achievement. This is as much for the process as the result. What do you want to learn about or do? If you enjoy reading, choose a book from a genre you do not usually select from or ask a friend for a recommendation. Join a dance class, do a puzzle, learn to play a musical instrument. Feel the buzz of learning and creating.

7: GIVE

While the desire to contribute positively to something beyond ourselves stems from a concern for others, there are benefits to our wellbeing too. We learn that it is immensely rewarding when we participate in an act of charity or engage in something bigger than ourselves: thanking someone, exchanging an understanding smile, participating in a community project enable us to connect with others and our environment, enriching their wellbeing and our own.

8: CELEBRATE AND HAVE FUN

Celebrations are fun, which is vital for our wellbeing. With life being a serious business a lot of the time, we all need opportunities to relax and enjoy ourselves. Try making a list of the activities you enjoy and pick a few to engage in over the summer. Have a picnic, go to the beach, eat lunch with friends, tell jokes and stories, and laugh. Smiling not only releases tension in our faces, it also lifts our mood.

9: SLEEP AND REST

As a practitioner you probably work long days and certainly carry a lot of responsibility. This can often result in unsatisfactory sleep, leaving you feeling ill-equipped for the following day. Experts in sleep hygiene encourage us to develop a rhythm and set of habits or rituals. These include no screen use before going to bed, lighting a candle or dimming the lights as we get ready to go to sleep.

Finding times to rest in the week is very important too. Opportunities to lay aside some of the busyness and engage in things we like to do. Time when there is no agenda and no pressure on us to perform – when we can simply be.

10: TALK

Some people get energy from interacting with others, finding that it helps them to process their thoughts, emotions and responses to events. Others do not need such external stimuli, finding extended conversations draining. However, there are times when sharing our thoughts and feelings with a trusted friend is important, particularly if we feel anxious. We build genuine friendships through trusted conversations, and such strong relationships help to build our resilience and ability to bounce back when life is difficult. Why not begin by asking a friend how they are and really listening to their answer. Showing such empathy will also help to nurture a relationship in which you might feel more comfortable sharing concerns too. Be wise in your choices, start small and see what develops over time.

This article was originally written for the teaching website **www.yellow-door.net**. *We are very grateful for their collaboration in creating it and their permission to share it.*

IN ALL THINGS CELEBRATE

by Talitha Fraser

I have this friend Dusk. She lives life large – she lives it full. When you tell Dusk good news, she'll cast her arms wide in flamboyant gestures and hugs while she squeals with joy and asks you question after question. There is no doubt that she shares in your hearts' joy when you are joyful and also in your pain when you are hurting.

In recent years, Dusk has had a rough road to walk – managing pregnancy and a new baby through family illness and bereavement taking their physical and emotional toll. It is hard to live big while living one day at a time.

I don't remember why she had them, nor what news elicited the joy but once as we caught up, she set off party poppers for every individual piece of good news.

Then we bought her a multi-pack.

It became a Thing. Through a hard time, she was able to celebrate many small moments of joy…a reminder that there were yet moments of celebration to find in the midst of it all.

My advice is this:

1. Pay attention to your joy and honour it

2. Get party poppers

MEDITATION

Making Moments

For this meditation, you'll need some stones or rocks.

I've always liked the stories of great leaders and pioneers from the Jewish tradition. People like Abraham, Jacob or Joseph made many mistakes and misunderstood Yahweh and his intentions for them often.

Wonderfully though, these people of faith found their way, formed nations, led people and provided hope for millions.

One of the things their tradition developed well was the ability to mark moments of significance. If their God saved them or something remarkable happened there was always a celebration, a festival, a sacrifice or a marker-moment to seal it. People were encouraged to remember with festivals like Passover which remembered the slave-people of Israel being saved out of Egypt.

Many of these figures make piles of stones to remember moments of importance. I like the idea that random people would walk along, see a pile of stones and think that something remarkable had happened to someone on this very spot. Celebration becomes communal.

For this meditation take some stones and make them into a pile.

Use this as a marker moment to remember the significant things that have taken you to the place that you are in your life. Maybe there's even a significant place to go and make this pile of stones.

Ponder the stones and ask why is this significant? What happened?

The other dynamic of these marker moments is that we have to walk away. No one stays there forever. How will you walk forward from this moment of remembering? What is it that is in this pile of stones which can give you the strength, resilience and courage to walk forward in your life with confidence.

What marker moments may be ahead of us in the future?

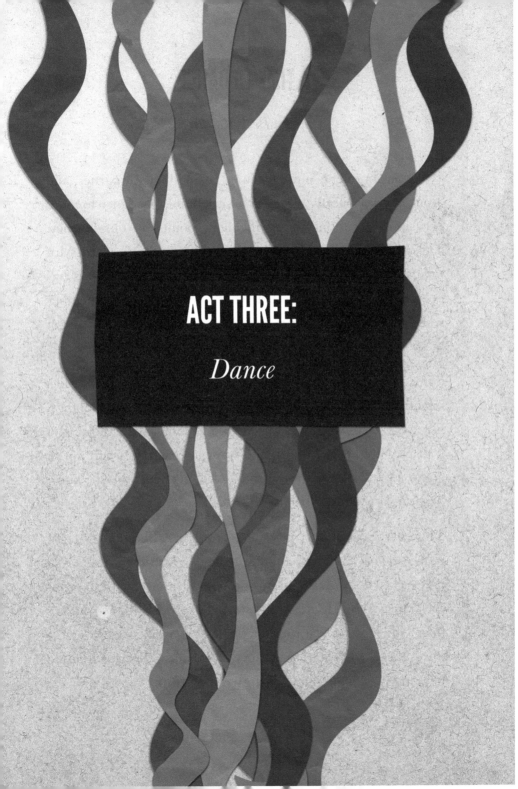

ACT THREE:

Dance

A TIME TO DANCE

by Beth Keith

We dance on nights out, we dance at weddings, at parties, and anniversaries. Mostly we dance to celebrate. We dance to mark occasions, occasions which highlight points on our journey. These moments to stop, and look back, and look forward. Moments to see how far we have come and to celebrate what has been achieved. To remember what's been hard, to remember what's been good, to dance the night away thankful that we got here.

Some celebrations simply mark out the passing of time, like birthdays. Some mark endings, like graduations, or beginnings, like weddings. Moments to dance and laugh with those who kept us going, who love us, and want to celebrate where we've got to. Friends who know what it took to get here and who know how the last year has been.

This year my daughter has started to dance. She is all of eight years old and has jigged about since she was little. She went to a dance class for a while, but this summer, she has started to properly dance. When I say, she has started to properly dance, I don't mean she has learnt a routine, or that the moves are perfect. I mean that she has started to move to the music, hearing it inside her, and marking it out in each twist and turn.

She has discovered her body, that she can move it and train it. She repeats the moves until her muscles know how to support her weight as she bends and twists. She spends hours dancing in the garden, sometimes with the music turned up loud, sometimes the music plays only in her head.

I could sit for hours watching her. It is one of those most beautiful things, watching her discover that her body is just that; it is hers. She moves as though this is her arena, her world, where she, and no one else, sets the time. She is discovering that she is in control of her frame, how it moves and shapes. How she can be in charge and given to the moment, setting the pace and also given to the rhythm around her, that she is flowing and still sure of her footing.

She is learning she is free, she is learning she is strong.

If you've watched Grey's Anatomy[15], you'll recognise that moment, when an episode is drawing to its close, when the trauma of the day's events has become too much, and all that is left is the invitation to dance it out. Perhaps it seems a strange response; to quit analysing, to stop reflecting, and regretting, and be lost for a few moments in music and movement. But after a day when the world has felt beyond our control, when we are reminded that we cannot keep each other safe, and where not everything we want can be fixed, perhaps sometimes the best response is just to dance. We could get medical and talk about the physiological response to trauma. How the body is flooded with adrenalin. How stress impacts on our bodies and minds. How movement can address these physiological changes, dissipate built-up adrenalin, and loosen tightened muscles. Our bodies are made for fight or flight or freeze responses, but our bodies are also made for rest, made to flow, made to dance. To be lost in movement and music, to mark out our space and set the pace, to remind ourselves that even when we cannot control the music around us, we are still free, and we are still strong.

We dance at our official celebrations, and of course the word celebration means to throw a party, but to celebrate can also mean to remember or mark an occasion. The word has close connections to another word commemorate, meaning to recall and show respect. Alongside our official celebrations, we may also have hidden anniversaries. Anniversaries of trauma and loss, events that have left lasting marks on us, and shaped the tread of our journey. Things we don't want to shout about, things that won't get written on any celebration card. Things which should be marked, and remembered, but celebration is not the right word. Perhaps commemoration says it better. To observe, to honour, to mark, and to remember. I haven't found the right word to sum up that feeling 'bloody hell, we made it through, we're still alive, and we're going to dance'.

A well-known poem in the bible begins:

For everything there is a season, and a time
for every matter under heaven.

A time to be born, and a time to die...

A time to weep, and a time to laugh...

A time to mourn, and a time to dance.[16]

We can see these words as separate and different. To be born and to die are not the same. To weep and to laugh are clearly dissimilar. But perhaps they are not opposites. Even in death, somehow, we are reminded that life continues. Through loss we remember the joy we knew. When we are most stretched, we find we are strong, and bravest when confronted by the thing we feared most.

That life can be simultaneously wonderful and achingly painful is something that deserves our respect, commemoration, perhaps even a little celebration. For grief and dance do not have to stand on opposite sides of a void seemingly impossible to cross. Turning, twisting, dancing, allowing our bodies to move in time, setting the pace, marking out the move. These things, seemingly meaningless, can help us to explore again what are bodies are capable of. That the body and mind can heal, that our spirit can know peace, and that strength can be felt.

Events of life can rob us of the belief that we are free. We can lose confidence in ourselves and in our ability to stand. We can lose faith in our power to set the boundaries. We can lose touch with knowing how to mark out our space and knowing how to live life. We may not always be able to control the music around us, but we can begin the dance, and rediscover our power to move and shape the world around us.

So, whatever you have to celebrate, or to commemorate, dance it out, mark the passing of time, respect what you have come through, and remember you are free, remember you are strong.

DRUM-THUD MISFIT

by Andy Freeman

Marquee madness,
Drum-thud misfit.
Requited gladness,
Womb-like mosh pit.
Home from home,
Black-dressed crowds,
Singing laments,
Shredding our shrouds.
Festival's heart,
Blood beating fast.
Here I'm a part,
Why won't it last?

NICKEL JUBILEE

(A Song of Ascents)

by Helen Dean

You are more likely to find me submitting
to oxygen at base camp than eagerly queueing
to summit Sagarmatha. Supine consumption
of Susan Cain's *Quiet* more my activity of choice
than subjecting myself to the hysteria of the arena.

Neither am I totally at home, quite yet, in an
arboretum of birdsong and pure fresh air
but I am learning to embrace this more and more,
along with savouring moments, no-caffeine drinks
and other such contributors to my well-being.

Ancient festivals all about joyful celebration:
first fruits, food, rest, outdoor togetherness,
assenting, ascending slowly, gradually, by degrees,
green places, thin places, always looking up,
tracing arcs of lost and found. Authentic after-party.

Dancing often, gratitude a daily dose. Come away
to sow in tears but reap in happy armful of sheaves,
empty-handed to clutching nascent twig of hope.
Celebration is not the two-by-two entering the ark
but the emerging as family out of it, dovetailing.

FINDING THE FESTIVAL

by Lucie Shuker

My daughter was born in mid-June, and I remember sitting on the sofa watching the coverage of Glastonbury as I held her. Maybe it was the hormones or the lack of sleep, but honestly, that festival has a mystical quality for me now. The low-sun glow reflected in performers' faces and the evening breeze lifting flags and banners, one by one like ripples on water. That big, big sky slowly changing colour. I still think about it.

We see a mirage when light rays bend, to create a displaced image of something in the distance. It comes from the Latin mirari, 'to look at or wonder at'. The displaced object is real – most often the sky, but what the distorted image represents is a product of our own interpretation. Holding my new-born daughter, I looked at thousands of people gathered to dance in a field as the sun went down and I saw…magic. I felt connected to them all. Every single one. We were all celebrating the same thing.

From a distance, and through the distortion of the multiple cameras and edited highlights, I have seen many other things in the heat of this particular spectacle. Face-painted girls in bikini tops, singing along to the words and sat high up on their boyfriend's shoulders. The synchronised bouncing of thousands of sun-glassed beaming faces. Spontaneity, joy and effortless life - come rain or shine.

It's a familiar trick of the light. The perception that this gathering is, was, or will be a piece of heaven on earth. In fact, it took me a while to acknowledge what my real experience of parties was. A sudden feeling of being completely alone in the crowd, of desperately wanting to hide and not being able to fake a smile any longer. When you realise the dark depths of the chasm between how you imagined this party might be, and where you actually find yourself, you come close to the mirage and it disappears. I kept my 18th and 21st birthdays about as low-key as possible. How can you host a party when you prefer the celebrations of your imagination? It wasn't until I turned 30 that I finally believed people would accept my invitation and possibly even have fun. Coaching myself as guests arrived, I decided not to care about whether anyone else was having fun. A psychological sleight of hand that worked pretty well.

The anxiety of celebrations is a recurring set piece in literature, on stage and on film. Whether it's a host whose angst infects the whole room, or a guest whose fears are writ large at a dinner party. There are those who care too much about what is happening, and whose concerns stifle any possibility of joy. That was me.

Then there are those who care too little. I recently watched Baz Luhrmann's adaptation of F. Scott Fitzgerald's novel and, man does that man know how to throw a party. Strictly Ballroom, Romeo and Juliet, Moulin Rouge and of course Gatsby itself. The scenes he creates are fantastical, conjuring a riotously noisy spectacle of colour and costume. But what he's particularly brilliant at, is evoking the chaos of the crowd. Fitzgerald described two of the main characters in his novel as 'careless people' who 'smashed up things and creatures and then retreated back into their money or their vast carelessness or whatever it was that kept them together, and let other people clean up the mess they had made.'[17] In each of these films, the lovers find connection beyond this chaos and carelessness. They retreat from various overwhelming scenes, as if coming up for air, and we see simplicity and authenticity set against the excess of the celebration.

I'm not surprised Luhrmann uses these set pieces in his story-telling. They thrill and dazzle. There's just something about a huge gathering that draws out our desires or fears on a grand scale. Take Michael Eavis, the co-creator of Glastonbury, who once said 'It's going to sound corny, but, well, it's a kind of utopia, really, something outside of the normal world we all live in'.[18] I'm sure I don't need to point out the many ways that festivals are not the utopia we might wish. But perhaps that's it. The larger the scale of the party, the more we can convince ourselves that it's a different world, with different rules.

When we come to a festival, we try to leave one world behind, in order to enter another. We hope that this pinnacle of our experience will be a gorgeous dream we enter as a reward for having gone to sleep. Of course, we never do really leave our lives behind. Our failed attempts at waking to a new world become apparent when the realities of day break into the dream. Anyone who has had a full-blown argument in the car on the way home or experienced violence on a campsite knows as much.

The distinction is not so stark of course. Most of us live in a kind of half-lucid dusk, between reality and fantasy. The mirage of the festival draws us in but we find we never quite reach it. Even our best experiences of the crowd or the music throw into relief how we feel about the rest of our lives. In 'The Festival Song', Pez writes that in light of the fun, it's weird that it's 'taken this long to shake last year's comedown'.

It's not weird at all Pez.

The way you do the party affects whether or not you experience a hangover.

Business academics coined the term 'festivalscape' to describe the cumulative effect of the intangible and tangible stuff of large celebrations in terms of 'consumer satisfaction'.[19] The programme, the physical environment, the reputation of the event: it all makes a difference. But they miss a fairly crucial aspect of consumer satisfaction - the consumer.

It's not all about what is happening externally because we bring ourselves to these events. Running from your real life, you may find respite for 48 hours but when it's time to go home, you're still the one you go home with. Some argue that festivals liberate by creating intense and playful experiences, where we get to 'try on' different possible selves. In these liminal spaces, these authors argue, the self and its relationships can be reconstructed.[20] I'm sure that's true, but perhaps not for everyone. I suspect that ultimately it is our inner world that creates much of the festivalscape we interact with, that opens or constrains possibility and that becomes memory to us. The mirage we see in The Great Gathering is one of our own making.

Henri Nouwen writes that:

> *Friendship and community are, first of all, inner equalities allowing human togetherness to be the playful expression of a much larger reality. They can never be claimed, planned or organised, but in our innermost self the place can be formed where they can be received as gifts.*[21]

With a gentle 'no' to the marketing gurus and business academics, Nouwen reveals that festivals, celebrations and parties are not 'delivered' on time or budget. The togetherness that they promise is only possible when we resist the mirage and the utopia. Instead, he invites us to allow a place inside us to be formed, where we have relinquished both our fantasies of community and our careless hedonism at the expense of others.

When this beautiful place is formed within us, we experience less of the come-down, less of the denial and less of a need to escape our lives.

One meaning of the word 'celebrate' is 'to honour…by refraining from ordinary business'.[22] While Michael Eavis delights in the possibility that Glastonbury is 'outside of the normal world we all live in', Nouwen nudges us toward making that normal world the place of preparation - to receive the festival as a gift. From the outside, it can look like festivals and parties belong to the young, the beautiful and the smooth-skinned. But if Nouwen is right, then celebrations are honoured most by those who have some faith that they are loved.

When this place is formed, to paraphrase Jesus, 'the festival of heaven is within you.'

MEDITATION:

Real-life Melody

For this mediation you'll need:

- ✓ A wooden spoon
- ✓ Everyday objects that can represent things in your life e.g. a half full glass of water.
- ✓ A sense of humour.

Our life is made up of everyday things. Sometimes it is hard to see them and their beauty. We take them for granted and they can merge into the background.

In this meditation I'd like you to think of up to ten things in your life that are important to you or that come to mind. They can be physical things like a house, they can be friends or family, or they can be things that are going on like a job change or a hope or memory.

Then go around where you live and find everyday objects to act as symbols or metaphors for these ten things. For example, a bowl could represent childhood, or a book represent learning.

Line these ten things up and get a wooden spoon. They begin to use the spoon to make a beat or melody. Don't worry if this is tuneful or not that doesn't matter.

Let all the everyday things speak to you about your life as you mess around with them.

What is the melody of your life right now? Happy or sad? Upbeat or slow? How do you feel about that? Make some decisions about what you value and what you might change or question.

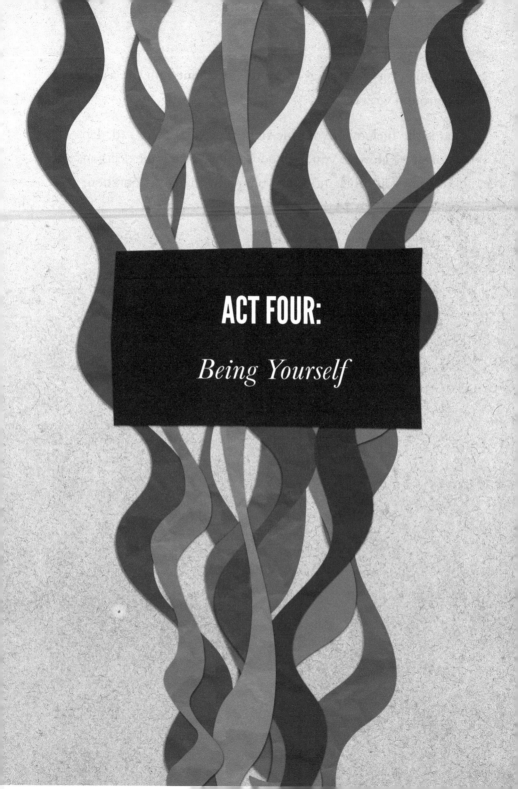

ACT FOUR:

Being Yourself

BEING YOURSELF: THE WELLBEING TRIANGLE

by Ben Harper and Andy Freeman

Many of the ideas and resources in this little book rely on what we at Space to Breathe call our Wellbeing Triangle.

Wellbeing is about thriving, not just surviving. When we had a think about what we thought being well or thriving is, we came up with three ideas – that it meant living well, living fully and living deeply.

This felt important to us. Being well is in essence about being to live well and healthily as ourselves. We are not required into a formula or to be someone else. Ben needs to be Ben well. Andy to live as fully and deeply Andy as possible.

But if that's being well – what are the ways we live well, deeply or fully? What are the ingredients for a healthy life?

At that point we needed coffee but thanks to some good hard thinking and some people who came before us, the Wellbeing Triangle emerged.

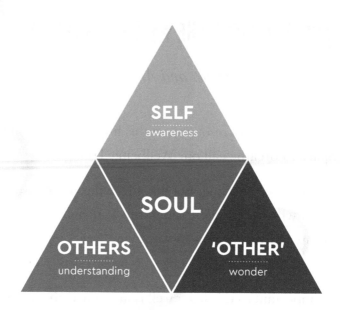

At Space to Breathe we use non-religious spirituality to help people increase their wellbeing. This isn't the only model or approach but it's one that we feel happy with and we think is often overlooked.

It tackles something important, that is often called the 'soul.' There's been various attempts in history to understand the soul and what it is.

The Oxford English Dictionary defines the soul as 'a person's moral or emotional nature or sense of identity'. In essence it's the 'non-material self' i.e. all the things within you that cannot be seen or quantified. It can cover awe, wonder, experiences explained or otherwise, unseen emotions or depth, unexplained tears etc. It's a dynamic that a spiritual approach to life recognises.

"It signals an interiority that permeates all exteriority,
an invisibility that everywhere inhabits visibility.[23] *"*

–Peterson (2005)

Having the Soul at the centre of an approach to identity and wellbeing brings significant value in our opinion. This approach aims to be non-religious and open to all beliefs and worldviews. But what we are saying is we believe the non-material core of ourselves when nurtured brings a sense of thriving and being well that is important for human beings.

This sense of soul is nurtured through connection and that is well represented by a Triangle. Triangles are geometrically balanced shapes that stand securely whichever way up they are. If one piece of the triangle was to be removed, the shape would become unbalanced and fall. This is true of our triangle – it requires all 3 parts to be present for the sake of balance and stability.

All parts of the triangle are connected. There is a relationship between them.

With 'Soul' at the centre our Wellbeing Triangle then seeks to balance three key areas of connection.

CONNECTION WITH OTHERS

We all have an innate need for this connection. Bowlby's work on early attachment in the 1970's has helped us to understand the profound impact that connection can have on the development of the brain. Connection actually makes the brain synapses grow.[24]

More recently, psychologists have understood more about the impact positive connections can have on those struggling with addiction and even suggested that addiction be addressed by increasing people's opportunities for connection.

Connecting well, fully and deeply with self will involve ideas such as vulnerability, kindness and understanding.

Essentially, we want to say that we need each other in order to be fully ourselves.

CONNECTION WITH SELF

We can only reveal to others what we know about ourselves and so connection with others is only possible when we have an awareness of self. This involves both having a sense of what makes 'me, me' (Identity) and emotional intelligence.

Daniel Goleman's[25] work on emotional literacy has shown that emotional intelligence (EQ) is a far better predictor of success than IQ. The ability to understand and manage our emotions is a vital part of our wellbeing.

Connecting well, fully and deeply with self will involve knowing your own strengths and weaknesses, being aware of your values (what makes you tick) and growing your own sense of sense awareness to perceive all these things.

To be "well" we will know ourselves a little more and be a little more comfortable in our own skin.

CONNECTION WITH 'OTHER'

If our connection with self is about realising our significance and growing our sense of esteem and value, connection with 'Other' might be about realising our insignificance in the context of the universe as a whole. Our wellbeing is supported by a healthy balance of the two.

'Other' can be described in a variety of ways. For people of faith 'Other' is often referred to as 'God', although it can also be about simply taking time to locate ourselves within something bigger than ourselves such as the world or universe as a whole.

Connecting well, fully and deeply with 'Other' will involve things such as wonder at the things around us and gratitude for the life we have.

In essence we'd like to suggest that in some way, we all need something outside of ourselves to be ourselves. Our engagement with "other" is a crucial axis of the triangle.

BEING YOURSELF

With these three axes in mind, the concept of being yourself and thriving as yourself can become a little more tangible.

I can grow and thrive in my sense of self if I take time to understand who I am, my values, personality and passions.

I can grow and thrive in my sense of connection if I take time to value and understand those around me, their impact on me and me on them. We are connected.

Lastly, I can grow and thrive in my sense of 'otherness' if I take to acknowledge and tend to those parts of me that are harder to quantify, harder to understand. My experience of nature, the sense of depth within me.

Then these three parts mutually nurture and grow each other. Finding myself in the awe and majesty of the world. Understanding 'otherness' more through the kindness of friends and strangers.

Oscar Wilde once said, "be yourself, everyone else is already taken.[26]" Wilde's wonderful and straightforward advice makes sense but is always harder to practice – how can I be me?

We've found the Wellbeing Triangle is a way to begin this journey. We can be shaped by so many things that happen to us but at our best, we thrive when we are allowed to be ourselves, not when we are squeezed into someone else's mould.

Be yourself. Go on. See what happens.

> *"I can be changed by what happens to me.*
> *But I refuse to be reduced by it."*

> *–Maya Angelou*[27]

TO THE MINI-ME

by Talitha Fraser

You, dear one
you exert so much energy
trying to be something other than
how you were made.
Rest. Rest and know
that you are loved, you are
a delight and I am
proud of you – just as you are.
Come, if you are weary
and heavy-laden and I will give
you a real rest, enfolded here.
Rest. Rest and know
that you are loved, there is no
one else you need to prove yourself
to or meet the expectations of,
there is no 'right' way or 'normal'.
Each person must walk their own path
and each is unique
– though your path may travel along
aside another's, it may not, or may
not always and it is not given to
you to know the way…

I know the way. It starts here.
Rest. Rest here awhile with me.
We can go on when you are ready.

SAFE PLACES

by Andy Freeman

If there's one barrier to being yourself that I know more than most, it's the fear of judgement. What happens when I'm truly me – what will people think? Dancing is one specific example of this.

As a 50-year-old I have no problem with dancing. I know my body moves poorly. I know I have the collective rhythm of a snail. The thing is that at 50 I don't really care. This is a freeing and releasing feeling.

However, I know I've not always felt this way. I remember the inter-school Disco with the girl's school down the road and sitting on a windowsill for the whole night, terrified that if I danced, I'd be laughed at. That night I cared a great deal. I was fearful.

Edmund Burke wrote "No passion so effectively robs the mind of all its powers of acting and reasoning as fear.[28]" Fear drives us, and fear restricts us. If I don't feel safe to express myself and be myself, fear will be the motivating factor.

This is sometimes the joy of a Festival. Have you noticed how people dress more expressively, are more open and adventurous at certain festivals? If a culture of expression is created and people feel safe, our fear diminishes, and we are more able to be ourselves. I find this fascinating. I doubt they'd be many days

I'd walk down Sheffield's Fargate area with flowers in my hair. I'd worry people would laugh. But at Glastonbury Festival, why not?

We are able to create cultures of safety that allow people to be expressive. Can we do that in our workplaces, in our schools and universities? What impact would that make?

In a 2017 Gallop Poll, only 3 in 10 employees strongly agree with the statement that their opinions count at work. Gallop calculated that if that increased to 6 in 10 it "could realise a 27% reduction in staff turnover, a 40% reduction in safety incidents and a 12% increase in productivity.[29]"

Gallop's findings suggest that if a workplace was a culture with reduced pressures to conform and with a reduced sense of fear, people would actually be more productive, achieve more in a more effective manner ... plus they'd be happy.

At Space to Breathe we've been deeply influenced by Any Edmondson's book 'The Fearless Organisation' (Wiley 2019.[30]) Edmondson talks about the concept of 'psychological safety' which makes so much sense to this idea of a culture of fearlessness.

In a psychologically safe culture, we are safe to share our opinions freely, disagree, be honest without fear, share about your life and feel released to listen to others.

This discovery has made a great impact at Google, which used it's Project Aristotle[31] to survey over 100 effective teams at the company – what made them work so well. The answer was psychological safety.

Teams can work well when people like each other, when people have key skills or when they socialise together. But the most important factor to an effective team is the freedom and safety to express yourself and be yourself. Amazing.

I love festivals and celebrations because the culture of them encourages joy, self-expression, dance and happiness. What would happen if more settings in our normal everyday lives expressed this same sense of psychological safety?

I'd like to find out.

Space to Breathe run regular seminars called 'Creating a Culture of Wellbeing in Your Workplace' sharing the concepts of psychological safety and working with organisations to build fearless cultures. To find out more visit **www.spacetobreathe.eu.**

MEDITATION:

Harbour

For this meditation you'll need your imagination.

Find a comfortable place to sit.

Get comfortable and relax each part of your body.

When you feel comfortable close your eyes and engage your imagination.

For this meditation I'd like you to imagine yourself on a small Fishing Trawler. It's been a long day and the nets have just been collected. Your catch is ok, but you know from forecasts a storm is coming and so you need to get to port.

On the horizon you see very dark clouds.

You pack everything quickly as the boat begins to make its way to shore. You can see the lights of the harbour, but they are bright with the darkness of the clouds behind you.

Slowly you make your way forward, but it seems like the clouds are moving faster. The wind is stronger, and the sea is stormy. The first crack of lightning rings out. It's going to be close.

Slowly you move forward.

Slowly the sea gets wilder.

You cross the entrance to the harbour. Feel the relief.

The sea relents a little.

Slowly you make your way to the harbour wall, tie up the boat and head to a local pub for shelter.

You sit by a fire, drink in hand and look out the window. The storm has taken hold.

Consider how safe you feel in the shelter.

Consider how unsafe you felt out at sea.

What makes you feel safe, fearless and gives you space to feel at peace?

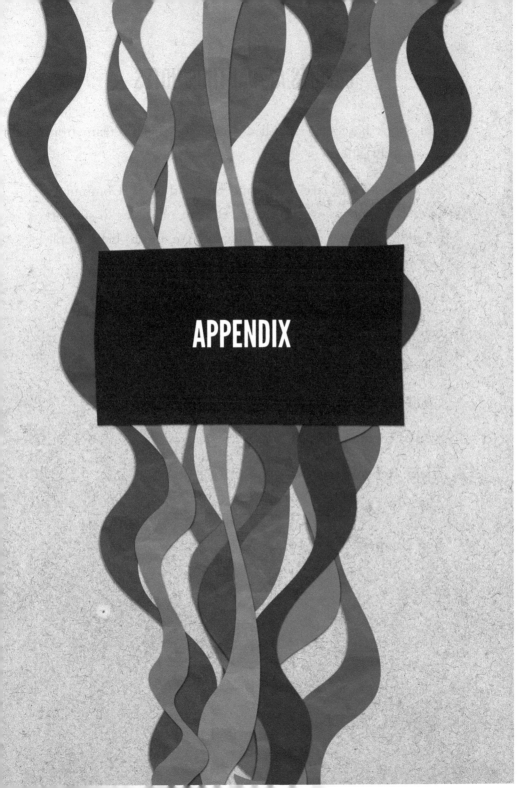

APPENDIX

CREDITS AND AUTHOR NOTES

This book has been compiled and edited by the team from Space to Breathe.

Space to Breathe are a growing Sheffield-based Community Interest Company who provide self-care resources to support people's wellbeing and mental health. We aim to help people live well, live fully and live deeply.

Check out **www.spacetobreathe.eu** for more.

Follow us **@space2breathe** on Twitter.

Follow us **@spacetobreathecic** on Instagram.

Contributions in this book come from:

Andy Freeman, *Founder and Co-Director,*

Nicky Redsell, *Co-Director,*

and

Ben Harper, *Educational Lead.*

We are so grateful to our guest contributors.

Richard Passmore is a Fresh Expressions Enabler in the Diocese of Cumbria. Follow him on Twitter **@richardpassmore**.

Martin Daws is a spoken word maestro from North Wales and a former Young People's Poet Laureate for Wales. He is also part of the band Baard. Follow him **@martindaws** on Twitter.

Beth Rookwood is a former British Skipping Record Holder and is also a Church of England Pioneer Vicar. She is building community in Northumberland. Follow her **@bethrookwood_** on Twitter.

Holly Crosby is a brilliant Sheffield-based coach and runs Simply You Coaching - **www.simplyoucoaching.co.uk** – you can follow Holly on Instagram **@simplyou_coaching**.

Talitha Fraser is a Melbourne-based New Zealand poet and writer. Check out her work at **www.thelightanddarkofit.wordpress.com**.

Beth Keith is Associate Vicar at All saints Ecclesall in Sheffield. You can find her on Twitter **@bethkeith_**.

Helen Dean is a Proost poet who recently published her first collection 'Double Entendre.' You can find her on Twitter **@HelenDean1850**.

Lucie Shuker is Director of the Youthscape Centre for Research. You can find her on Twitter **@lucieshuker**.

HELPFUL NUMBERS AND INFORMATION

However, we are always aware in our work that sometimes more help is needed, and that self-care isn't always the totality of what we need. If these exercises raise any concerns for you about your own health or that you know you're already struggling we'd suggest you take some simple but important steps to get further help.

✓ Please talk to someone about how you feel. Most advice suggests this is always the first and most important step. Friends, family or professional services all fit the bill here.

✓ Please do get help from your Doctor or GP. If that feels like a tough step to take, services such as the Samaritans and Mind are a great help. We've posted a few contact details overleaf.

✓ Please do keep yourself safe. You are wonderfully valuable, and we think you're amazing. When considering what to do and how you feel always make sure you're safe and you're making choices which prioritise your own health.

If you'd like any help at all, you can contact us, and our team will reply as quickly as we can. Use **info@spacetobreathe.eu** and we'll get in touch as quickly as well. Our team aren't Doctors or Counsellors so it may be that we need to connect you with someone we know and trust who can help you, but we'd be happy to hear your story and offer what help we can.

We've found that the following organisations are wonderful and incredibly helpful if you need additional support.

ANXIETY UK

Charity who support people diagnosed with an anxiety condition.

Phone: **03444 775 774**

Website: **www.anxietyuk.org.uk**

MENTAL HEALTH FOUNDATION

Provides information and support for anyone with mental health problems or learning disabilities.

Website: **www.mentalhealth.org.uk**

MIND

Campaigns on behalf and supports people with mental health problems.

Phone: **0300 123 3393**

Website: **www.mind.org.uk**

SAMARITANS

Confidential support for people experiencing feelings of distress or despair.

Phone: **116 123** (free 24-hour helpline)

Website: **www.samaritans.org.uk**

YOUNG MINDS

Information on child and adolescent mental health. Services for parents and professionals.

Phone: Parents' helpline **0808 802 5544** (Mon to Fri, 9.30am to 4pm)

Website: **www.youngminds.org.uk**

CRUSE BEREAVEMENT CARE

Phone: **0844 477 9400** (Mon to Fri, 9am to 5pm)

Website: **www.crusebereavementcare.org.uk**

BEAT

Supporting those struggling with eating disorders.

Phone: **0808 801 0677** (adults) or **0808 801 0711** (for under-18s)

Website: **www.b-eat.co.uk**

RELATE

The UK's largest provider of relationship support.

Website: **www.relate.org.uk**

ENDNOTES

[1] Mind 2016

[2] https://www.theguardian.com/education/2019/apr/16/fifth-of-teachers-plan-to-leave-profession-within-two-years

[3] This guide was created for Tramlines but is designed to be flexible for other settings. It is available for download at https://www.spacetobreathe.eu/stories/2019/7/15/tramlines-festival-free-wellbeing-guide.

[4] Guardian, October 2018 'Is gratitude the secret of happiness/'

[5] Sirois/Wood 2017 Gratitude study lowering depression in Chronic illness populations - https://www.ncbi.nlm.nih.gov/pubmed/27786519

[6] Wood/Froh/Geraghty 2010 - https://www.ncbi.nlm.nih.gov/pubmed/20451313

[7] Kate Fox 'Watching the English' Hodder & Stoughton 2004

[8] Rumi 'Selected Poems' Penguin 2004

[9] ibid

[10] Maya Angelou, Celebrations: Rituals of Peace and Prayer, Viragao 2009

[11] Meister Eckhart, Selected Writings, Penguin 1994.

[12] Tony Buzan quote sourced online.

[13] (www.nhs.uk/live-well/eat-well/)

[14] See mindful.org

[15] Grey's Anatomy

[16] Ecclesiastes 3:1-4

[17] F Scott Fitzgerald 'The Great Gatsby' 1925

[18] Michael Eavis, Glastonbury Festival 1995, cited in McKay 2000.

[19] Lee Y., C.Lee, S.Lee and B.Babin (2008) 'Festivalscapes and Patron's Emotions, Satisfaction and Loyalty.' Journal of Business Research 61 (1) 56-64.

[20] Kim and Jamal 2007 Wang 2000

[21] Nouwen, H (2000) Reaching Out

[22] https://en.wiktionary.org/wiki/celebrate

[23] Eugene Peterson, 'Christ Plays in ten Thousand Places' 2005 Eerdmans

[24] We used John Bowlby & Attachment Theory by J.Holmes 1993.

[25] Daniel Goleman 'Emotional Intelligence: Why it Can Matter More Than IQ' Mass Market Paperback – 12 Sep 1996

[26] Oscar Wilde anecdotal.

[27] Maya Angelou 'Letter to my Daughter' Virago 2004

[28] Edmund Burke from Amy Edmondson 'The Fearless Organisation' Wiley 2019

[29] Gallup Poll 2017 from Amy Edmondson, ibid

[30] Amy Edmondson, ibid

[31] Project Aristotle from New York Times article - https://www.nytimes.com/2016/02/28/magazine/what-google-learned-from-its-quest-to-build-the-perfect-team.html